Ethical Issues in Dementia Care

Bradford Dementia Group Good Practice Guides

Now under the editorship of Murna Downs, this series constitutes a set of accessible, jargon-free good practice guides for the carers of people with dementia. Reflecting the group's commitment to the person-centred approach to dementia, the series draws on both experience in practice and the latest research in the fields of dementia and dementia care.

other titles in the series

Social Work and Dementia
Good Practice and Care Management
Margaret Anne Tibbs
Foreword by Murna Downs
ISBN 1 85302 904 1

Primary Care and Dementia
Steve Iliffe and Vari Drennan
Foreword by Murna Downs
ISBN 1 85302 997 1

Healing Arts Therapies and Person-Centred Dementia Care
Edited by Anthea Innes and Karen Hatfield
ISBN 1 84310 038 X

Training and Development for Dementia Care Workers
Anthea Innes
ISBN 1 85302 761 8

of related interest

The Simplicity of Dementia
A Guide for Family and Carers
Huub Buijssen
ISBN 1 84310 321 4

Perspectives on Rehabilitation and Dementia
Edited by Mary Marshall
ISBN 1 84310 286 2

Food and Mealtimes in Dementia Care
The Table is Set
Grethe Berg
Foreword by Aase-Marit Nygård
ISBN 1 84310 435 0

Bradford Dementia Group Good Practice Guides

Ethical Issues in Dementia Care
Making Difficult Decisions

Julian C. Hughes and Clive Baldwin

Jessica Kingsley Publishers
London and Philadelphia

First published in 2006 by
Jessica Kingsley Publishers
116 Pentonville Road
London N1 9JB, UK
and
400 Market Street, Suite 400
Philadelphia, PA 19106, USA

www.jkp.com

Library of Congress Cataloging in Publication Data
Hughes, Julian C.
  Ethical issues in dementia care : making difficult decisions / Julian C. Hughes and Clive
Baldwin.
    p. cm.
  Includes bibliographical references (p.   ) and index.
  ISBN-13: 978-1-84310-357-8 (pbk. : alk. paper)
  ISBN-10: 1-84310-357-5 (pbk. : alk. paper) 1. Dementia--Patients--Care--Moral and
ethical aspects. 2. Medical ethics. I. Baldwin, Clive, 1962- II. Title.
  RC521.H84 2006
  174.2'983--dc22
                                    2006006215

British Library Cataloguing in Publication Data
A CIP catalogue record for this book is available from the British Library

ISBN-13: 978 1 84310 357 8
ISBN-10: 1 84310 357 5

Printed and bound in Great Britain by
Athenaeum Press, Gateshead, Tyne and Wear

To Ann and Peter Hughes,
Patty and Sarah Rebekkah
with gratitude and love

Contents

Figures and Tables

Preface

The aim of this book is to help carers of people with dementia. In the main we are thinking of non-family, formal carers, but the book draws in large measure from research with family carers and our hope is that it may be of interest to all those who work, live and care for people with dementia. We hope it will help carers not only to recognize the ethical issues involved in caring for people with dementia, to understand how to deal with difficult (ethical) decisions and to gain some confidence in making such decisions, but also to be aware of the need to involve other people appropriately when the decisions are too difficult.

The aim is not to teach carers how to be experts in medical ethics. However, we are keen to encourage the idea that all carers, inasmuch as they become expert at dealing with difficult decisions in relation to dementia, gain expertise in ethical matters. Being more reflective about this would, we hope, improve decisions made with or for people with dementia. In other words, our approach is underpinned by the thought that much ordinary care involves an ethical component, even if it is not recognized as such. Our hope is that increased reflection on the ways in which ordinary care is given should enhance that care, whether or not the reflection is regarded as 'ethical'. Ethics is all about treating people with dementia well.

The book stems from research with family carers of people with dementia. Clive was the main researcher in that study, funded by the Alzheimer's Society, whose support we have acknowledged. We have not, however, acknowledged our collaborators in that research, who have been well disposed to our use of some of the material from the research in this book. Professor Tony Hope, then the Director of Ethox, led the research project. More significant for us, perhaps, has been his kind encouragement and support over many years. We have both undoubtedly benefited from his tremendous expertise in the field of medical ethics. Professor Robin Jacoby contributed his wealth of both clinical and research experience in old age psychiatry to the project. More personally, during Julian's higher training in old age psychiatry Robin was his supervising consultant for two years, an experience that continues to provide inspiration and for which he remains grateful. Sue Ziebland imparted her understanding of qualitative research methodology and contributed a deep enthusiasm and expertise in medical sociology to the project. To Tony, Robin and Sue we offer grateful thanks, not only for their collaboration, but also for their friendship.

The research team, however, was broader still. It included Sandra Bemrose, Meg Gilpin and Carol Green, consumer monitors from the Alzheimer's Society's Quality Research in Dementia (QRD) panel. We benefited enormously from their perspective and contribution to the design and progress of the project. But the project would not have been possible without the cooperation of the carers up and down the United Kingdom who gave their time so willingly and who discussed their (sometimes painful) experiences with openness and generosity of spirit. We shall remain grateful to them. Many of them agreed to the recordings of their interviews being used on DIPEx, a charity-run 'patient experience' website (www.dipex.org). The research project led to a publication by the Alzheimer's Society (Baldwin *et al.* 2005) intended for family carers, with many sources of further information. A more academic preliminary account of its findings is recorded in Baldwin *et al.* (2004).

We should also like to thank Jessica Kingsley and her team, who have been patient and supportive publishers. Helen Ibbotson and, more recently, Jessica Stevens have acted in a kindly and considerate way as our editors and have guided us during the production of the book. We also benefited from Christine Firth's astute copyediting and Sara Millington's careful proofreading. We are grateful to the whole team. The diagrams in Chapter 2 were executed, with his usual alacrity, by Luke Hughes, to whom lashings of thanks. Various students have read through a draft of the book and we are grateful to them for their helpful comments. They were Jane Barrington, Georgina Cox and Clare Hunter. Emma Hughes also kindly commented on chapters of the book. We are very grateful to Agnes Muse who typed the original drafts with her usual humour and efficiency.

The book would not have come into being, however, without the invitation of Professor Murna Downs, the series editor. Having extended the initial invitation, Murna has continued to be encouraging and always positive in her comments. With her typical candour, she may deny that she has had much else to do with the book. However, knowing and talking with her as both a colleague and friend continues not only to be a source of pleasure, but also to widen our field of view. Through her deep appreciation of the issues for people with dementia and their carers, she challenges our patterns of practice in ways that are wholly beneficial. We are enormously grateful to her. However, all of those we have thanked bear no responsibility for any deficiencies in the thoughts expressed in the book, which are entirely our own.

Research on dementia is understandably dominated by the scientific explanation of the diseases concerned and their treatment. At the coalface, however, the quality of the lives of people with dementia are dominated by the individual interactions experienced day by day and minute by minute. Many such interactions involve carers making decisions about people with dementia: decisions about how to keep them safe, what they should eat, and whether they should be treated this way or that. These decisions carry ethical weight and should be made with care and thought. We hope this book will contribute to an atmosphere in which this can be the case.

Julian C. Hughes
Clive Baldwin

Acknowledgements

We are enormously grateful to the Alzheimer's Society who funded the research project that lies behind this book. All of the quotes from carers (and some of the anecdotes) are taken from interviews conducted by Clive Baldwin during the research, which was undertaken at Ethox, University of Oxford, between 2001 and 2004. The quotes are used with the permission of the participants in the research, although the names have been changed throughout the book. Julian C. Hughes would also like to acknowledge the generous support of the Wellcome Trust, which (in 2003) funded a short-term fellowship for him to carry out research into the conceptual basis of quality of life in dementia.

Chapter 1

Making Moral Decisions
From consequences, duties and principles to conscience

INTRODUCTION

Morals are messy; ethics is everywhere. These are the two themes we wish to stress in this chapter. Before explaining what we mean by them, it is worth saying where these themes will lead us. We shall see, first, the extent to which morality is not as neat and tidy as some theories suggest, and second, that ethical decisions are commonplace: we make them all the time. This leads to the conclusion that from day to day we often have to make difficult decisions for which there is no neat and tidy theory to help us. In short, we live in a messy world. Our job – which we cannot avoid – is to find our way through the messy world day by day. The hope, of course, is that we can do this successfully and even with some satisfaction.

However, perhaps we have already jumped ahead of ourselves by not defining what we mean by 'moral theories' and 'ethical decisions' (see definitions overleaf).

> **Moral theories** – systems or structures of thought and belief that help us to decide what is good and what is bad.

> **Ethical decisions** – decisions about what it might be right or wrong to do.

Moral theories give us ways of understanding what might be a good thing and what might be a bad thing. They can provide a framework for the ethical decisions we have to make. We would certainly not wish to be too critical of these moral or ethical theories. They have, after all, been developed by some of the world's greatest thinkers and they reflect deep-seated beliefs. But in the busy world of dementia care, as in other areas of practical life, applying such theories can be a problem. In order to show the strengths and the weaknesses of such theories, we shall consider two of them very briefly (consequentialism and deontology) and discuss an approach that is derived from these theories (called principlism). Our intention is certainly not to try to give a full account of these moral theories (see Gillon 1986); in fact, we really wish to get them out of the way – but we need to say why.

CONSEQUENTIALISM

The word 'consequentialism' conveys a simple message: if you want to know whether an action is right or wrong, look at the consequences of doing or not doing it. Now, this can be a very sensible way to decide whether or not what we want to do is good or bad and, indeed, people do tend to think in this way. For example, one husband caring for his wife, when asked about why he had decided to lock the doors and windows in his house, replied:

it appeared to be the lesser of the two evils because to let my wife out was a very dangerous thing because that was at the time when she was going off, she was setting off on a journey of 180 miles to where her parents had lived, which, obviously, there were a lot of dangers with it. And there was a suicidal attempt. She tied herself to the gates of an old cemetery, a disused cemetery on a cold day. She could speak at that stage and when I did find her and brought her home I said, 'Whatever were you thinking of?' and she said, 'I want to die.' So locking doors, locking her in, was the alternative to possibly letting her go out to commit suicide.

Another carer talked about how she decided on whether or not to tell her mother with dementia the truth. She took into account whether her mother would be distressed:

> I would say that it's good for everybody if we can all tell the truth but I think that we have to recognize that the truth sometimes does more damage than a lie, and is better withheld. You've always got to put the person first. Never mind what your own thoughts are or your own feelings, you've got to put yourself in their shoes and the effect on them is what you're concerned about. So a little white lie is sometimes a very good thing.

There are problems, however, with looking at consequences only in order to decide what is right and wrong. An often-used example is the case of the runaway railway carriage that is hurtling along a line and is going to kill five workmen if it is not stopped. You are standing next to someone and you can stop the train by pushing him or her onto the track. The consequence would be one death as opposed to five. From a purely consequentialist point of view, it looks like the right thing to do would be to push the person. However, most of us, even if the certainties were 100 per cent, would not entertain such a thought. Pushing the person seems in itself wrong, whatever the consequences. The point is that looking at the consequences, at what follows, takes our eyes off the action itself. We may end up doing something terrible in order to do something good. Some people feel that this is such an awful idea it makes this way of thinking completely unacceptable. They might put it thus: the end *never* justifies the means.

This brief description of an extremely influential moral theory shows us already one problem (see definition of consequentialism below): ethical theories get argued about, and always have been argued about, so how can we rely on them when we are faced by difficult decisions in our daily work?

> **Consequentialism** – to decide if an action is right or wrong by looking at its consequences (e.g. will doing it make people happy or sad?). *But* does the end always justify the means?

DEONTOLOGICAL (DUTY-BASED) ETHICS

The even grander word 'deontology' means something just as simple as consequentialism. Deontological theories suggest that if you wish to know whether to do something, you should not ask, 'What are the consequences?', but rather, 'Is it my duty to do this?' The word deontology implies – and can be replaced by – the words 'duty-based'. So, we might say that we have a duty to protect innocent human life. In health and social care, for instance, people talk about a 'duty of care'. The idea is that once you become responsible for someone, you have to care for him or her, not because of the consequences, but simply because it is your duty to do so. In fact, the consequences of caring for someone may be quite bleak: caring is stressful, time consuming, sometimes un-rewarding, potentially harmful (think of lifting someone), expensive and may in the end seem pointless if, for instance, the person dies. Still, we accept the duty of care. It seems to be a good thing in itself for one person to care for another. For some family carers, this 'duty of care' comes in the form of their marriage vows:

> Well, I've put it [being a carer] down to the fact that I have a strong sense of duty, generally and that's confirmed by my contact with other carers... If you've married somebody, you're partners for life: you look after them and they look after you, so if anything goes wrong you look after them, it's as simple as that... And more importantly if somebody *needs* you then you should respond.

As you might have guessed, however, there are arguments against duty-based ethical theories. For instance, some have argued that we always have a duty to tell the truth (whatever the consequences). The schoolboy, Tom, knows that the consequences of telling the truth and admitting that he smashed the window will mean that he gets into trouble, but we would still argue that Tom has a duty to tell the truth. However, to use an old example, if in the Second World War you happened to know that the Jewish family of Anne Frank were hidden in a house, if asked by the Gestapo, would you have had a duty to tell them the truth? In other words, sometimes the consequences of an action are much more important than the nature of it (see definition of duty-based theories below). Who cares about the duty to tell the truth if telling the truth leads to something abhorrent?

Duty-based theories – to decide if an action is right or wrong by deciding whether it is the sort of thing you ought to do as a duty (e.g. we might think we normally have a duty to save a person's life if it is in our power to do so). *But* can we really just ignore the consequences of our actions?

We ended the section on consequentialism by pointing out that ethical theories are themselves constantly argued about. Now we see that this problem is made worse, because there are different ethical theories that sometimes seem to argue in different directions, so how do we know which one to choose? (The arguments for and against numerous different ethical theories are very well presented in Hope, Savulescu and Hendrick 2003.)

PRINCIPLISM

One way to get round the problem of choosing between ethical theories is to plump for 'principlism'. The idea is that whichever ethical theories we might prefer (and there are other theories than the two we have mentioned), they tend to support certain principles. So, instead of learning all about the moral theories, we could simply stick to the principles and this should ensure that we always do the right thing.

The common principles are these (Beauchamp and Childress 2001):

- *Autonomy*: people should be able to decide what they want to happen or be done to them.

- *Beneficence*: we should try to do good to the people we care for.

- *Non-maleficence*: we should try to avoid doing people harm.

- *Justice*: people should be treated fairly and equally.

These are sometimes known as the 'four principles of medical ethics', but others can be added, such as:

- *Fidelity*: we should always tell the truth and be truthful.

- *Confidentiality*: we should always keep the information we have learned in confidence about people we care for safe and private.

Although these are referred to as principles of *medical* ethics, they are principles that are used in everyday life too. Here for example, Walter, a family carer, talks about respecting the person's autonomy:

> I think in the early stages of the illness there was always a tendency to take over. So, for example, if he couldn't tie his shoelaces, instead of just letting him try for a bit longer, the natural thing is to say, 'Come on, let me do it', when in fact I've now learned that what I should have been doing was allowing him to do it in his own way however long it takes because…that's, if you like, respecting their independence and their autonomy.

Another carer, Harold, mentioned how, with the idea of doing good in mind, he made decisions regarding:

> things like coming out of the choir. Well, basically from what I learnt from [the day centre] was, 'Is this any benefit to the person? And if it isn't, well then there's no point in putting them through it any longer'. She came to village things for ages, people knew how to handle it. And as long as I felt it was doing her some good we kept going.

A third, Harvinder, discussed doing good and avoiding harm:

It [medication] would certainly have to be monitored very carefully to make sure it is a correct medication because we all know that if we have something for a month and it's not doing any good or it's doing you harm, the side effects or something, it has to be changed.

The trouble with these principles, however, is that they can conflict and sometimes pull us in different directions. For instance, a doctor might be certain that he or she can make a person better; so in accordance with the principle of beneficence (i.e. doing good to people) the doctor ought to do whatever will make the patient well. However, respect for autonomy (i.e. the principle that people should choose for themselves) might mean that the person's right to refuse treatment should be respected. Put like this we might be tempted to say, 'Well, it seems fairly obvious that the person's wishes are crucial, so it looks as if autonomy always trumps beneficence'. But should this always be the case? Let us consider some specific case examples.

Case example: the man with a bad headache

Mr Able has had a bad headache for over 24 hours. He goes to the doctor and after a few tests is reassured that there is nothing sinister going on. It is just a headache. The doctor offers him some stronger painkillers, but he refuses and says he is able to put up with it.

Conclusion: The doctor must respect Mr Able's autonomous decision not to have more tablets.

Case example: the psychotic inspector

Detective Inspector Nye, who has always been a capable and successful police officer, starts to develop paranoid delusions. He is not sleeping because he feels he must keep watch from his bedroom window. He is firearms trained and he seeks permission to take a gun home with him. He is encouraged to see a doctor, who wishes to have him into hospital for investigation and treatment, but he denies there is a problem.

Conclusion: It is more difficult to respect the inspector's autonomous wishes. It sounds as if he has a serious mental illness, which may reflect an underlying physical condition that could be treated. In order to do good (beneficence), perhaps he should be detained against his wishes under the Mental Health Act (HMSO 1983).

Case example: the pregnant phobic woman

Mrs Angst has had an unremarkable pregnancy. Normally she is fit and well, but she has an overpowering fear of needles. She goes beyond her due dates and there are worries about the baby's health. Eventually the obstetrician wishes to perform a caesarean section to get the baby out safely. But Mrs Angst is too worried about the need for a drip and she refuses to have the caesarean.

Conclusion: Such cases have gone to court in the past because they are so difficult to decide. Mrs Angst's right to make decisions about her body (as required by respect for her autonomy) is in direct conflict with the need to do the best thing for her and for her baby (the principle of beneficence) and the need to avoid harm befalling either of them (non-maleficence).

Case example: living with dementia

A man was caring for his elderly wife at home and his wife would get up in the middle of the night and go downstairs and sit in the cold living room. The man used to wake up and go downstairs and try to persuade her to return to bed where she would be warmer and more comfortable. The woman used to refuse so he would 'semi-force her to go back to bed'. He knew that this was against her wishes, but also that going back to bed would be better for her than sitting in the cold, lacking sleep.

These examples show that autonomy is not always the winning principle (see definition of principlism below). The conflict between principles shows that there must be something else at work, there must be some other way of deciding between the principles when they clash.

> **Principlism** – to decide if an action is right or wrong, the principles of medical ethics should be applied; the principles give us a way to discuss dilemmas in clinical ethics and thereby ought to help guide action. *But* sometimes the principles conflict and then we need some other way to decide between them.

MESSY MORALS

This section takes us back to where we started. The discussion of ethical theories (consequentialism and deontology) and principles shows what we meant when we said that morals are messy. Moral theories and principles do not provide neat and tidy answers. Actually, they can sometimes make matters more complicated. It may be perfectly true that a paternalistic doctor has always acted beneficently. Sure of himself, Dr

Paternalistic used just to get on with it and act in his patients' best interests. Now he has to check what the patients think and want. This makes him hesitant and uncertain. Sometimes he ends up being persuaded to do things because his patients want him to, but which he feels may not be for the best.

Alternatively, Dr Autonomy is a great advocate of patient choice and always feels that the patient's autonomy should be respected. In many instances this ensures that better decisions are made, because the patients' views are heard and taken into consideration. But then she is confronted by the psychotic policeman (in the second case example in this chapter) and the idea of him being able to take a gun home is very frightening. Moreover, it starts to seem not only unreasonable, but also unacceptable, that he should be able to refuse assessment and treatment.

The truth is that adopting an extreme position will always make the person prone to criticism from some moral theory or other and so, generally speaking, the better thing to do is to pick and choose between principles and moral theories. To pick from different doctrines in ancient Greek times was to be *eclectic*. But there are two things about being eclectic. One is that it is messy. There is no nice, neat system. In one case we pay attention to the consequences and decide it is better to treat the person with dementia with some medication; in some other case we ignore consequences and focus instead on, say, the duty to tell the truth (e.g. about the diagnosis), even if it is painful.

The second thing about being eclectic (picking and choosing) is that it almost sounds as if you can do whatever you want. You just find the moral theory or principle that suits you. The trouble with this is that it seems to undermine the very reason for having a moral theory in the first place. These theories and principles were meant to tell you what to do;

now it turns out you have to decide what to do by picking and choosing between the theories and principles. It seems that the theories and principles give you a way to *describe* why it is you do what you do, but they do not *dictate* what to do in the first place. This is why we said earlier that we really want to get these theories and principles out of the way, because they are often presented as if they will give a definitive answer, or as if they are all that is required to deal with moral dilemmas. To say we wish to get them out of the way is to overstate the case because, as we have already suggested, they reflect profound thoughts and beliefs. It is just that, in the real world, they do not usually give us neat and tidy answers. The moral field is decidedly messy and we must navigate our way through it carefully, whereas these moral theories and ethical principles can send us hither and thither.

CONSCIENCE

But what then do we use to help us navigate our way in the messy world of morals? How do we, in fact, decide about good and bad, right and wrong? Our suggestion will be shocking to many moral philosophers and medical ethicists, partly because it is an old-fashioned idea and one that can easily be criticized. Our suggestion is that, by and large, *conscience* guides us.

The obvious response to this is to say that conscience is not much of a guide, it is far too subjective (see definition of subjective moral theories on p.27. Surely conscience can say almost anything we want it to? Probably many perpetrators of genocide have been able to claim that their consciences were clear: they were acting under orders, defending themselves, making the world safer, or better, or whatever. But who cares what their consciences said? They took part in the mass killing of innocent people (see for example Lifton 2000).

Does this not show, therefore, that conscience is not to be trusted?

Well, our response is to point out that there are two ways of thinking of conscience. First, there is the little voice – as it were – in our heads that tells us what we should be doing or not doing. Perhaps I promised to ring the wife of someone I am looking after who has dementia, but my shift is now finished and I am keen to get home. There is that irritating thought, or voice of conscience, however, reminding me that I said I would ring her. I know I cannot relax, or feel at ease with myself, until I have spoken with her. My conscience is pricking me, suggesting what I have to do.

Now this way of thinking of conscience may seem fine – the right thing to do is to pick up the phone – but it is precisely this sense of conscience that can go wrong. What if I am working in a nursing home for people with dementia and my conscience starts telling me that the right thing to do is to pick up the pillow and suffocate Mrs Dean? Just because the voice inside my head tells me to do it, does this make it right?

Subjective moral theories – what is right and wrong is decided on the basis of my individual inner re-flections and feelings (i.e. these theories are like our tastes).

Objective moral theories – what is right or wrong is decided on the basis of outer facts and shared values (i.e. these theories are like social rules).

The second way of thinking of conscience is to see it not just as something I concoct for myself, but as something more objective (see definition of objective moral theories above). The key thing is that conscience should be *informed*. We acquire an informed conscience through education and up-bringing. Actually, other moral theories and principles can contribute to the informing of conscience. But conscience is not generally thought of as being a particular moral theory. It is more a part of the messy moral world. It is itself eclectic. What is clear, however, on this view, is that conscience can go wrong. Someone can be *mis*-informed, but this is difficult to imagine on a huge scale because we all tend to be brought up in a world that shares a host of similar concerns. This is why we hope that those who have knowingly committed genocide have had some sleepless nights: otherwise it suggests that the objective notion of conscience can be overridden on a big scale. Nevertheless, it is also possible that on the basis of a correctly informed conscience, a person might make some slips in terms of the interpretation of it. There may be all sorts of reasons for this, from illness to a lack of will power. But this, at least, supports the possibility that conscience can have an objective element to it, even if it occasionally goes wrong.

Anyway, beyond what we have already said, we do not need to analyse 'conscience' here.[1] Rather, we simply wish to suggest that, in the hurly-burly of the messy moral world, in actual fact conscience does usually act as our guide to what is right and wrong. The important (more objective) point relates to how our consciences have been (in-)formed. This will not ensure there are no arguments. Actually, it might be said that the arguments are part and parcel of how we inform our consciences. We think it is right to tell patients what we think might be wrong with them, say, but it makes sense to discuss this with people (especially with patients) to test whether this view is fair. We might come to see that it is not always a good thing, or we might be even more strongly persuaded that what we tend to do can be done *in good conscience*. Being open to the possibility that we might be wrong is an attitude of mind that a good conscience might suggest.

We criticized other moral theories on the grounds that they might not act as good enough guides. Conscience, on the other hand, is just the guide that most of us are aware of and, where there are arguments between people of good conscience, these arguments (as long as they are reasoned and rational) are a way of moving us towards the right answer. It is not that we say we know what this is in any certain way, but we can feel our way towards it by open, tolerant discussion, navigating our way through the messy world of morals.

Case example: conscience and finance

One carer, Simon, reported that although he did not have power of attorney for his partner, he (Simon) sorted out all the expenses. This sometimes meant that he wrote out cheques and had his partner sign them, even though his partner may not have realized what he was signing. Simon was aware that this was possibly illegal but did not want the involvement of the Court of Protection:

> The-day-to-day running of all the expenses I sort out anyway and it's working very well. But I had a word with the solicitor who deals with a lot of the Alzheimer's Society things and he said to me, 'You're in a very dangerous situation.' I said, 'Well, maybe I am, but I'm not prepared to do anything about it unless I'm forced to.' And if anybody can come to me and say you're doing the wrong thing I shall say, 'No I'm not.' Not, you know I can satisfy my own conscience about what I'm doing and that's all that matters to me.

Case example: conscience and assisted suicide

Another carer, Jaroslav, expressed the opinion that requests for assisted suicide might be made because the person making the living will might not know what Alzheimer's is, or what it involves, and thus might be making an ill-informed request. Jaroslav continued:

> I'd be hard pushed in my own conscience. I mean, say for instance my wife had had this Will and she said that [she didn't want to live], I don't know whether I could do it or not. I might *want* to carry out her wishes but whether I could. I mean I can't even kill a mouse! So I would be hard pushed in that direction I think. Very hard pushed.

In both these cases the thing to note is that the carers refer to their consciences as, in a sense, the judge of what is right or wrong. Their immediate appeal is to the little voice in their heads that tells them they are right to do (or not do) whatever it is. But the suggestion is that this justifies their actions or decisions in a way that is compelling; that is, the voice of conscience seems to be decisive as if it has external authority: they cannot go against it. An ethicist trying to change the person's mind, therefore, might use a variety of arguments. In the end, however, the arguments will be successful only if the ethicist is able to gain a purchase on the level of all that has informed the person's conscience. This may be more or less difficult depending on how well formed the person's conscience is, which will depend on a whole raft of external factors reflecting education, social and cultural values, and so on.

In the chapters that follow, one of the things that we see ourselves doing is to present information, different viewpoints, facts and values that will help to inform consciences. Of course, all of us already have well-formed consciences. What we shall be doing is laying out the moral landscape around dementia care. This landscape will always be seen from a different (and unique) perspective. For the same person things might look different on two occasions, because we change and our different experiences change the way in which we see things. We shall be drawing on the experience of family carers of people with dementia in order to think about how we, as formal or professional carers, look at things. Seeing our way through this landscape, understanding why a particular path is right, or what makes another approach bad, is to inform our consciences. It is to store up shared views that will then guide our own difficult decisions. It is not that we make these decisions alone, solely relying on our own individual consciences, it is that an individual conscience is informed by common, shared understandings and practices. This common, shared world of practices is the messy, eclectic world of morals. It is this that we shall explore.

ETHICS IS EVERYWHERE

One of the things we shall find as we explore the messy world of morals is that ethics is everywhere. Clinical practice, caring for people, is by its nature an ethical enterprise. There is almost no decision we have to make in dementia care that does not involve a question of right or wrong. At the level of clinical practice these ethical decisions are sometimes very obvious: shall we put a feeding tube through Bill's stomach wall now that his dementia has progressed so far that he cannot swallow? But some more mundane clinical decisions can also be ethical decisions. Should we give Jessica, who has dementia, a tablet to calm her down at night? There are empirical questions here (i.e. questions that could be answered by facts); namely, will the tablet work and what will be its side effects? But there are also ethical questions: is it a good thing for Jessica? How do we weigh up its good and bad points?

However, not all decisions are clinical decisions. Many of them will relate to ordinary day-to-day care. Should we talk to Bill and Jessica as we pass them in the corridor? The everydayness of ethical decisions (which would fall under the concept of microethics used by Komesaroff 1995) is abundantly clear in the lives of family carers for people with dementia. In the extracts that follow, from an interview with Marguerite, a woman who was caring for her husband who had dementia, we see a broad range of issues:

> Ethical issues. There were, money related things. My husband, he'd always had very good jobs, very responsible jobs and he'd invested fairly wisely and when I took over power of attorney when he was getting in a real mess, it's managing to keep things going, or whether I should keep them going. And whether I should perhaps sell them or change them…
>
> Charities are another area. For a long time any charity that came through the post, [my husband] would look at it and he would read it very carefully and say, 'Oh, this is a good cause', and he would write off, like normally put a ten pound note in it. One charity that just *will* not leave him alone and he sent off a cheque for £147 to them. Maybe it is a worthwhile charity but I've only ever heard of them when they've written to him! I don't know anything about them and so now I've got control, I no longer send to that charity. But I have to think well hold on, he's joined the British Heart Foundation, National Children's Society I think and the Lifeboat. Now you know, I feel maybe I should carry on with subscriptions to those…

For a long time I was actually hiding his letters because when I was at work I never knew what was happening you know when, when I got home so I used to have to try and waylay the postman and actually take the letters to work until I'd vetted them. Things I recognized I let him have...

Another thing, I mean his politics and mine are totally different and I feel that I should let him carry on supporting his political party, you know, I mean he wrote off £200 to them when they wanted their election campaign. So yes that, that's something which he would have done when he was well...

We made wills when we got married but I have changed mine so that I can safeguard my children's interests. I felt really bad about that because initially we both left everything to each other and if we'd both died together, everything would be divided eight ways. But at the moment I say, I have changed my will so that any cash assets I have in my name will go to them and half the house will go to them. So I've done that, again I felt bad about that...

Health. The 'biggy' for me now is resuscitation. When he started going for respite care they ask you whether you feel any heroics in terms, in case of collapse or anything and then I, I didn't even consider anything other than 'Yes, do what you can.' But now I'm beginning to think, 'Well hang on, what's his quality of life. If he has a major stroke or a major heart attack he's going to be vegetating.' For a man who was always so fit and proud of his fitness is this a good thing, you know will he, would he actually want to be treated like he'd have to be treated?...

I feel I have to make decisions for him and speak for him not only to professionals but also I need to keep the family informed and also I'm finding I have to tell other people now, you know I mean my friends know the situation. Some of them are very understanding; some of them don't seem to be quite so patient or willing to visit any more. But you know how much do I share with people?...

And also he's been a bit inclined to shoplift once or twice. So again I felt I need to tell people, 'Yes my husband has dementia, I'm sorry he's taken this, you know, here it is back, is that OK?' So yes, you know, how much information should I share with people?...

And the other thing is like sort of day-to-day management, dealing with his post, fielding phone calls. And sometimes it was more convenient to give him a different sort of time, if he hasn't got his watch on and I want him to hurry I might push the clock forward a bit in his head and my head.

CONCLUSION

We have ended with talk of day-to-day management, which chimes with our theme that ethics is everywhere. Many of the day-to-day decisions that have to be made in dementia care turn out to have an ethical component: not just whether or not we use a feeding tube, but how we talk to people. We have also pushed the idea in this chapter that morals are messy. There are no easy solutions and, more importantly, no straightforward ways in which to find the answers to our moral dilemmas. As we have seen, the major theories and principles of medical ethics can conflict. Our shocking suggestion has been that we should pay more attention to conscience as our moral guide. Conscience has an inner aspect to it: the little voice in our minds. But informed consciences are justified in the world, where values are shared and disputed. In this light, the disputes are seen as in-tellectually healthy, because they challenge the formation of conscience. In this book our aim is to survey the difficult decisions that have to be made in dementia care and offer a variety of approaches as a way of challenging our attitudes. As in this chapter, we shall rely on the real stories of carers to raise issues. However, we shall also endeavour to develop an approach to ethical issues in dementia that fits with the experience of practice.

NOTE

1. It may seem that we are 'copping out' by not discussing conscience any further and in fact there is little written about it because it is so unfashionable. However, Hudson (1967) gives a very clear account. There are other ways of thinking about conscience. For instance, the idea that there might be something more objective behind the notion of conscience is seen in the medieval distinction between *conscientia* and *synderesis*. These notions are very clearly explained and discussed in a posthumously published essay by McCabe (2002).

Chapter 2

Being True
Relationships, empathic understanding and communication

INTRODUCTION

This chapter is about relationships, but these are based on understanding and communication. We shall use the specific example of truth-telling. A lot of what we say in this chapter is about being true to people and about being open to their perspectives. Before we move on to think more specifically about the relationships that surround people with dementia, it is worthwhile thinking about relationships in themselves.

RELATIONSHIPS AND PERSONS

One thing is clear, a relationship always involves at least two people. If we start to think about this, we can immediately see that the simplest relationship involves three things: there are two people, but in addition there is the connection between them (see Figure 2.1). Of course, the connection does not exist without the people and the connection does not have to exist: it is not inevitable that Bob and Mary will have a relationship.

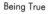

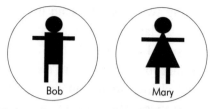

Bob and Mary as independent individuals

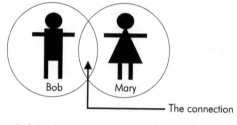

The connection

Bob and Mary in relationship

Figure 2.1 Individuals and interconnectivity

So we can think just about Bob and we can think just about Mary. If we cut all the connections that might surround Bob and Mary, we end up with the solitary individuals. That also means we end up with two unrelated perspectives: on the one hand, there is how Bob sees the world; on the other hand, there is how Mary sees it. Now, the first lesson we wish to draw from this simple analysis is that the individual's point of view is very important. To understand a person, and to understand a person's relationships, we need to see things from the person's point of view. Being able to do this is also called empathy: that is, putting yourself in his or her shoes.

While it is true that Bob and Mary can be considered as individuals without connection, does it really make sense to think of them without any relationships at all? In other words, while Mary and Bob might not have a relationship with each other, it is highly likely they will have *some* relationships.

We are making two types of claim in saying this. First, there is an empirical claim (that is, one that may or may not be true and can be tested for), namely that as it happens, most people are in connection with someone else. Second, there is a more conceptual claim, which can be put like this: for a person to be a person is for him or her to have relationships. In other words, part and parcel of what it is to be a person is for the individual to be connected with others. This is an *in principle* claim. It does not require an experiment to prove whether or not it is true.

Of course, we *could* do an experiment. Some people have tried to imagine what it would be like to be Robinson Crusoe, alone on an island. Yet this is not quite right, because there is no doubt that Robinson Crusoe is a person for two reasons. First, even though he has no human relationships (until Man Friday comes along), he had human relationships before he was shipwrecked and these must have contributed to making him the sort of person he is. For instance, he might have been taught by his parents to be self-reliant and practical. Second, even without human relationships, Robinson Crusoe still has relationships, for instance with animals, but maybe also with other aspects of nature; he approaches these relationships from a human perspective, the one gained when he did have human relationships. So there are reasons for thinking that Robinson Crusoe is inevitably a fairly sophisticated sort of person for whom relationships count.

No, the correct experiment would have to be one in which the human being never had *any* human-like relationships at all, as in the case of Kaspar Hauser in German folklore (Herzog 1975; Wassermann 1983). Kaspar Hauser was brought up in a small locked house in a forest, never seeing who or what it was that provided his sustenance. We might wish to call Kaspar Hauser a person, but he was certainly emotionally and intellectually deficient. Nevertheless, as soon as Kaspar Hauser was left in the town square of Nuremberg, relationships started to develop as others encouraged him to adapt to the real world.

The point is that, in actual fact, it is difficult to conceive the correct experiment to prove or disprove the 'in principle' claim. This is partly because the result of the experiment is called into doubt as soon as it ends and the individual, however deficient, comes into contact with the real world of relationships; but, in any case, the claim was *in principle*. The claim is for a person to be a person, as a matter of principle, is for the person to have relationships. We cannot disengage the person from his or her connections.

This idea is not new, of course. The Greek philosopher Aristotle referred to humans as social animals. Over a thousand years later, the English poet John Donne wrote that 'no man is an island' (Donne 2000, p.344). In the 1920s, the Jewish writer Martin Buber referred to the person by using the expression 'I–Thou'. In other words, to understand the person properly is not only to understand a single person, an 'I', but also to appreciate the person in the context of relationship, as an 'I–Thou'.[1] And this notion had a significant impact on the ideas of Tom Kitwood (1997), to which we shall return.

So there always is an Other. The significance of this is that the person (Bob or Mary) cannot, in fact, be thought of without thinking about his or her connections. The consequence is that when I put myself into someone else's shoes, when I see the world from their perspective, I also see the person's connections. Let us now put this in terms that are often used by medical ethicists. All individuals are to be treated as being autonomous (see Chapter 1), but actually none of us is totally independent. Part of what it is for us to be persons is for us to be connected by our relationships. These relationships are always unique, so the perspective is always unique. But more than that, it is not just that we are made up (at least to some extent) by our relationships, it is also that we inevitably depend on those relationships. We depend on our husbands, wives or partners for emotional support, but we also depend on the greengrocer for our fruit and the bus driver for our transport. In short, we are autonomous *and* interdependent. As such, we have a unique point of view, but it is a view that involves our connectivity, our interconnections.

Persons – can be considered not only as individual autonomous agents, but also as mutually dependent and connected by relationships.

As indicated above, the person can be understood in different ways, but – as we have argued – one crucial aspect of being a person is that we form relationships and this natural ability seems to be essential to us. Not only is it essential because it keeps us well balanced as human beings, but also it is essential 'in principle' because part of what it is for us to be persons is for us to have this essential connectivity to others. Now, how does all this relate to dementia?

DIFFERENT PERSPECTIVES AND EMPATHY

One feature we have already touched on is the importance of perspective. To understand other people is to understand their perspectives. This will include their perspectives on events.

Case example: understanding the other's perspective

Akanke had been admitted into hospital in order to be assessed. Because of the emergency surrounding the admission, Akanke had not had time to pack many clothes and her neighbour offered to go and collect these from Akanke's flat. Akanke, however, refused to give her the keys because she did not want anyone going through her things, even though this neighbour had been looking after her for quite some time and Akanke herself could not go to the flat to collect the clothes herself. From the perspective of the carers, this was a practical issue of collecting clothes. From Akanke's point of view it was an invasion of her privacy and a curtailment of her freedom.

To act in good conscience (see Chapter 1) is partly to make sure we have seen the landscape properly. To do the right thing we need to be able to see the views, the perspectives, of the various people involved. In the case above, seeing Akanke's point of view was necessary in order to try to help her. Acting ethically, doing the right thing, involves finding a route through these different perspectives. Our analysis of relationships helps, even if it also reveals how complex things may be. We said earlier that understanding people included understanding their perspectives on events, but it also involves understanding their perspectives on relationships.

When we think of the person with dementia, where the ability for the person to act entirely as an individual, autonomous agent (making decisions and life choices completely independently) can become limited, what we see is a degree of dependence. The extent to which we are connected to other people becomes emphasized. If Bob develops dementia, he becomes dependent on Mary perhaps. But even 'in his prime', Bob was already connected by his relationship with Mary. Moreover, even 'in his prime' that relationship – if it were a good one – would have involved mutual dependence. Mary needed Bob – or at least was supported by the relationship – and Bob needed Mary – he too was supported by their relationship. Now that he has dementia that dependence has been increased.

Let us say that into this relationship comes their family doctor. One thing she has to do is understand her patient, Bob. But to understand him she must understand his relationships: they constitute, or help to make up, his standing as a person. You might say that the doctor must understand where Bob stands. However, where he stands is in relationship with Mary. Bob has a perception of this relationship and it is important for the doctor to realize that the relationship, the connection, has a history. Part of the strength (or weakness) of their relationship will depend on the different experiences they have shared that have increased (or decreased) the connection between them.

Of course, the doctor's involvement instantly creates a new relationship; in fact, two relationships, one with Bob and one with Mary. As the doctor makes decisions concerning Bob, these will inevitably have an impact on Mary. The possibilities are countless. One decision may ease the burden on Mary, perhaps by increasing the connection between the doctor and Bob. For example, the doctor may wish to encourage Bob to attend a day hospital on a regular basis for a while. But Bob may or may not want the connection with Mary to be lessened; or he may or may not wish to have such a tight connection with the doctor, whom he hardly knows and whom he worries about in case she intends to take away his independence. Another decision may leave Mary feeling excluded (perhaps she feels she is losing her connection to Bob).

Doctors (and other professionals), therefore, need to move with care as they negotiate these relationships. It is easy to get things wrong, as explained by Richard:

> At the time, the neurologist, most of my in-laws and almost everyone else told me that my wife should not be told what the true problem was. I now disagree emphatically with that. It removed any scope for me to combine with her to combat the problems she had. It also meant that I had to do a variety of pretty awful things by subterfuge. I had to remove her driving licence, her bank cards at different stages, chequebooks – all kinds of things like that – without being able to tell her the reason I was doing it. This, of course, caused an incredible amount of bad feeling, and ruined our relationship in many ways. Even though I was the person that she depended upon, she didn't like me, I think, for most of the remaining time, because of all these things that I'd done. I was the obstacle in her life in many ways.

Similarly,

> So finally, nearly two years after my husband had originally gone off sick, we arrived in this clinic where they specialized in unusual dementias and my husband went through a whole series of tests. He was admitted for three days and the diagnosis was made that it was frontotemporal degeneration/Pick's disease. So we were faced with a situation where having previously been told it was probably Alzheimer's, there was then a huge question. So I asked the consultant, if he felt it wasn't Alzheimer's, what he felt it was and his answer to me was wholly dismissive. Basically he had given his opinion, time would tell. I was told, 'Only time will tell'.

Well, that threw up the first problem, which was, if it may not be that then why, having been told by two different doctors that he shouldn't drive, my husband's concern was, 'Why should I not be allowed to drive?' The consultant said, 'Would you mind leaving the room while I discuss this with your wife?', which my husband did. The consultant discussed it with me, called my husband back into the room and said, 'Well, as a result of talking to your wife, I must now recommend that you don't drive'.

Now that threw the onus wholly on to me and my husband perceived me as the wicked wife who had persuaded everybody that he was unfit to drive; and that I think did more harm to our marriage than anything has ever done before or since. My husband and I were at each other's throats. We were destroying each other with this awful driving issue. And I don't think that man had any possible concept of what he [the consultant] was doing to us as a married couple, by not accepting the responsibility of having to make a decision as a professional and stick by it. The whole onus was thrown on to me and it was devastating. It harmed us for months and months and months. So that really could have been avoided, and I believe should have been avoided.

What we see in the real world is, of course, complex. Some people have only one relationship, but many people have all sorts of different relationships. Bob and Mary may have a son, Joe, so his connections and perspectives also come into play. Again, these connections can be various. Some sons are very close to their parents; some are more distant. A son may be closer to one parent or the other. The relationship may be viewed differently by the son and by the parent, e.g. it may be valued hugely by the parent but of little concern to the offspring, or vice versa. Someone, like the doctor, steps into these networks of interconnections (see Figure 2.2).

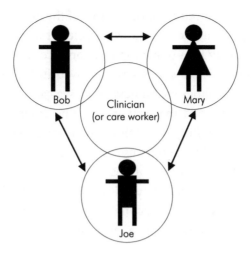

Figure 2.2 Individuals and interrelationships

Actually, things are more complex because the doctor, by establishing these relationships, is, to some extent at least, altering the relationships between the other people involved (see Figure 2.3).

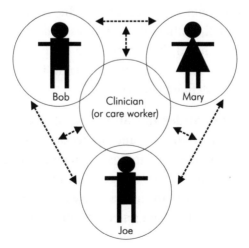

Figure 2.3 Interrelationships and interdependency

So far we have concentrated on the role of the doctor in these relationships. But the person who enters the network of connections may be a home carer or someone working in a nursing home, where she is now involved in looking after Bob. The possibilities are endless. Now we can see what we meant when we said that acting ethically, doing the right thing, involves finding a route through different perspectives. To do what is right – and let us admit that this will often be instinctive, that is, people will just do what seems to be the best thing at the time (i.e. they will act 'in good conscience') – will, at its best, involve acting in a way that enhances relationships in a way that, in a sense, makes the connections better.

There are, however, two points to make. First, although we have said that people act instinctively, there is still the moral requirement that their instincts – or their consciences – should be informed. Part of the point of this chapter is to emphasize the extent to which this involves understanding people in the context of their relationships and under-standing their perspectives. As carers (of any sort), to do good we must enter these contexts in an understanding way. We cannot presume we understand the connections, the importance of the different viewpoints and their histories, unless we have heard their stories and really tried to stand in their shoes. That is, a basic demand is for empathic understanding (defined below).[2]

> **Empathic understanding** – the ability to step into the shoes of another and appreciate what might be meaningful (i.e. how things are understood) by seeing the world (including the person's relationships) from the perspective of the individual, where this perspective also has a history and reflects a culture and society.

Second, the idea of 'enhancing relationships' or of 'making the connections better' needs some comment. This sort of enhancing or making better is not always comfortable for everyone concerned. It may even be painful. In a paradoxical way, the relationship may be enhanced by the connection being made looser. It may be that Bob's tight ties to Mary are causing them both problems. It may be that Joe's wishes, e.g. that Mary keeps Bob at home for as long as possible, reflect his perspective and his needs, but may be a disaster for Bob and Mary. (Equally, it could be that the doctor's view that Bob should be in long-term care is simply askew, because she has not seen the extent to which Joe would wish to support his mother in her wish to keep Bob at home.) What will be enhancing or helpful will, once more, need to be negotiated and tested out through empathic understanding. It is not inevitable, however, that the result is stronger connections. For our connections also have depth and, it has to be said, they can also be unhelpful, even malignant. This is another notion, to which we shall return.

TRUTH-TELLING

For now, however, let us consider some specific examples around the notion of truth-telling. The example of doctors telling patients the truth about the diagnosis is now a fairly obvious one, although it is still true that this does not always routinely happen in dementia care (Bamford *et al.* 2004). The inclination either to tell the truth or to withhold it can be regarded as showing similar concern for the patient. Furthermore, in both cases this concern can centre on the nature of relationships. Thus, the doctor (along consequentialist lines and in order to avoid harm) does not tell the patient the diagnosis because it might upset her and, in any case, her son has said that he does not want his mother burdened with this news. But this will place some sort of stress on their relationships. The mother knows, perhaps, that something is not right with her; yet she is surrounded by people who do not seem willing to tell her the truth. Alternatively, because the doctor has strong beliefs in autonomy, in the patient being able to make decisions, she is told the diagnosis (perhaps the doctor feels a strong sense of duty to tell the truth). This may be very helpful, because she can now make plans for the future. However, she may become depressed at the news, showing that the son was right and making the therapeutic relationship between the doctor and the family harder to negotiate. On the whole, however, openness and honesty are helpful to relationships, whereas deceit and dishonesty are unhelpful.

Case example: truth-telling

Alana was concerned about her mother, Marie, who had become really quite forgetful and was 'filling in the gaps' with accounts of things that had never happened. For instance, Marie had lost her coat and had told Alana that she had been burgled and the burglar had taken the coat. According to Alana this was when she faced her first ethical dilemma:

> I wasn't sure if I should tell her the truth or not, that was really difficult. I knew the truth would be painful for her, I knew my mother was the type of person who wants to know the facts as they are. My relationship with her had always been based on trust. To deceive her would be far worse. I opted for the truth. I never thought it would be a smooth ride but it was simply *awful*. When she asked a direct question I was careful to tell her the truth only if I was 100 per cent certain. If I were not I would say, 'I don't know.'

The above example, which involved nothing so grand as the truth about the diagnosis, but only the truth about a mislaid coat, nevertheless entailed a painful decision.

What about a man with dementia (let's call him Ian) who is persistently found to be having sexual relations with another resident in a home, called Liz? Helen, Ian's wife, does not know. Should she be told? One obvious answer is that she might well discover anyway, so she should be told. But the news may be extremely upsetting to Helen. On the other hand, not to tell her means there is dishonesty between the staff in the home and Helen, who may then start to feel that something is being covered up. She may gradually feel less secure about Ian being in the home.

Again, in general it would seem likely that honesty is the best policy. There may be several sorts of difficulty. There needs to be some honesty over whether this relationship is after all a good thing for Ian and Liz. Is it entirely mutual? How would they feel about the relationship if they realized what they were doing? Even if it were thought to be good for Ian and Liz, if it were not something Helen could accept, difficult decisions would have to be made. Can one of them be moved to another part of the building? Might one of them have to leave the home? What would be the consequences of such a move?

At issue is the very nature of relationships for the person with dementia. There is no clear-cut right or wrong answer without knowing the details of the case. What the details allow us to do is to put ourselves in the shoes of the people involved to see their different perspectives. To ignore any particular perspective (Liz's view for instance) is to fail in terms of empathic understanding. The answer is likely to be one that emerges from an honest discussion and consideration of the different viewpoints. Under the circumstances, the decision is likely to be painful for someone. Attempting to view the different perspectives with empathy, however, and taking into account the background ethical norms and laws, will be the way to make the decision with a clear conscience. An example of a relevant ethical norm might be the need to give Helen's views a good deal of weight, given her standing as Ian's wife for 45 years. Relevant laws might be the laws that relate to mental incapacity or the guidance around vulnerable adults. A further point that emerges from considering such a case, however, is the importance of good communication.

Relationships are maintained by good communication: between family members; between professionals; between professionals and patients or users; and between professionals and carers. It could be said that the quality of the communication might have a direct impact on whether something is right or wrong (see our discussion of communicative (or discourse) ethics in Chapter 5). Take, for example, the experience of Ged being asked by a research centre whether he would donate his wife's brain for research:

> But the thing that was perhaps the cruellest experience that I had was when my wife was actually in the hospital for the assessment and they had told me it was best, she would get better care in a nursing home. And it was at the period that I was looking for the nursing home I received a letter through the post at eight o'clock on a Saturday morning, a cold letter asking *me* to donate my wife's brain for research.
>
> At that period it was just *totally* bad timing again through lack of communication between everybody. The research centre were not aware that my wife was being assessed, and that it had been advised that she go into a nursing home. But the letter was very, very cold, there was

no lead into it. It was just a very cold letter asking me to donate my wife's brain to research. I found that a very, very cruel, bitter experience.

The lack of sensitive communication and lack of consideration of the feelings of the carer impacted directly on the ethics of the request for brain donation. In other circumstances, at other times, and done differently, the request could have been entirely appropriate. And it might even have provided an opportunity for some good to have come from what, for Ged, was an horrendous situation. As it happened, the request caused considerable distress.

COMMUNICATION AND CARING

Thinking about relationships led us to think about communication and the idea of empathic understanding as a way of ensuring that the different points of view of the people involved in relationships are considered. But the idea of empathic understanding brings us round to think about the person in more detail. It also takes us back to the two points we have left hanging in this chapter so far.

You will remember we spoke of Buber's notion of the 'I–Thou', of the person in relationship. This was an idea picked up in relation to dementia (Kitwood 1997). Kitwood saw 'dementia sufferers' first and foremost as people with dementia. In fact he used to write of the *person* with dementia, rather than the person with *dementia*. He was keen to stress that a person had to be understood as a social being. We are what we are, to a considerable extent, because of our relationships. This led Kitwood (1997) to the idea that people with dementia might be made worse if the quality of the care that surrounded them was poor. In fact, to pick up the second point we left hanging, he referred to 'malignant social psychology'. That is, a person might be surrounded by such negative influences – in terms of the social environment – that he or she might be made worse.

Here is a trivial example, but one that can be common-place.

Case example: communication and empathic understanding

Bob, who has dementia, does not understand why he has been left in a residential home for respite for a week. During the morning of his first full day he asks several members of staff when he is going home. He is booked in for seven days, but several of the members of staff tell him that he will not be there long (which leads him to believe he is going home later that day). However, he quickly forgets this and asks the same question again. Eventually staff ignore the question. Bob becomes agitated, starts walking around and finds the outside door, which is locked. He pulls at the door and eventually a member of staff comes to take him back to the lounge, saying he should have a cup of tea. Once there, he is left alone and he starts to pace again, finds the door and again pulls on it. Once more he is encouraged back into the lounge for a cup of tea. This cycle of events is repeated. Finally, Bob is becoming quite frustrated. A new member of staff comes on shift and tries to encourage him back to the lounge again. By this time the sun is going down and Bob is sure Mary would want him home soon. Bob has had enough and when the staff member gently lays a hand on Bob's arm, Bob swings at him and catches him on his face. Because Bob is now agitated and aggressive, he is given some of the medication written up by the doctor specifically in case this sort of thing should occur. Bob now feels odd and unsteady and, still unsure where he is, he tries to leave his bedroom later that night and falls over, banging his head.

In this story it is the social environment that leads to a worsening of Bob's state. Our purpose here is not to set out everything that Kitwood (1997) said about malignant social psychology. It is worth noting, however, that Kitwood argued that the social environment, the quality of care provided to people with dementia, could be improved. He suggested this might have the opposite effect to that described in the story: it might actually make the person with dementia more able to deal with things and understand what is going on when the social environment is encouraging rather than discouraging. How this might be done is also well documented in the work of Professor Steve Sabat, a psychologist in the United States, who has shown how good communication and empathic understanding can help to sustain the person with dementia (Sabat 2001).

CONCLUSION

Our purpose, however, is to make a point about ethics. It is this: although big ethical decisions sometimes face doctors and carers of people with dementia (we shall discuss some of these in Chapter 3) and although some difficult decisions can be quite dramatic (e.g. what to do about the sexual liaisons of Ian and Liz), many of the very ordinary day-to-day decisions are also ethical. These are often to do with our relationships and the quality of our communication. Spending five minutes with Bob, not hesitating to re-explain things, engaging his interest in a genuine way, not misleading him, finding him meaningful occupations, these might all be small matters but they can make the difference between doing him some good and doing him harm. In each case, it is the quality of our connections with Bob that are improved and, if all that we have suggested in this chapter is true, improving the relationships that surround him is a way of enhancing his standing as a real person.

NOTES

1. Martin Buber's (1878–1965) use of the notion of 'I–Thou' has theological connotations that we are not exploring here. However, a fuller exploration of the importance of relationships in connection with dementia from a theological point of view can be found in Allen and Coleman (2006).

2. The notion of 'empathic understanding' can be found in the work of Karl Jaspers (1883–1969), a psychiatrist and a philosopher, who worked in Heidelberg in Germany. His work on psychopathology (the illnesses of the mind) continues to be very influential. See for instance Schwartz and Wiggins (2004).

Chapter 3

Concerned to Treat

INTRODUCTION

This chapter deals with issues that relate to treatment. Before considering some specific treatment issues, we shall pause to reflect on the very idea of 'concern'. This will be the background against which we then discuss consent and capacity. We spend some time on these notions because having the right approach here underpins the sort of treatment decisions we discuss later, when treating or not treating can seem equally problematic for all concerned. It is worth also reflecting that 'treatment' can mean very ordinary things – the fleeting interactions of everyday life. In turn, this will take us back to the theme of Chapter 2, because once again we shall be talking about relationships and understanding.

CONCERN AND THE HUMAN CONDITION

Let us imagine we are standing somewhere. In a sense, where we stand will decide how 'concerned' we are. So, if we were standing on a thin ledge on the side of a mountain, we might ordinarily say that we should be very concerned. If we were standing, alternatively, in the middle of a beautiful garden surrounded by friends and family we might, again in that ordinary way, say we should be very unconcerned. We wish to use the word 'concern' in a different way to argue that *where* we stand does not really alter how 'concerned' we are. Rather, we are concerned simply because of the sort of creatures we are. We may be more or less concerned, but that simply reflects *how* we are as human beings. It does not reflect *where* we are so much as *who* or *what* we are.

In our special sense of the word, to be concerned is part of being human. To lack concern in this sense is just not to see what it is that we are. Equally, although this might be the wrong reaction, if we see too clearly that essentially we are 'concerned' beings, we might become over-anxious. So what is this special sense of the word 'concern'?[1]

It really implies that to be a human being involves being connected and interconnected. It means that, wherever we happen to be standing, we are (by our nature) linked to the world. As beings of this sort, the world has meaning for us – even if we are depressed and think everything is meaningless – in a way it does not for other creatures. The world for us, as human beings, is not simply a world of things. It has a significance for us. To put it another way, we are engaged by the world, whether we are engaged by its barrenness and brutality or by its beauty and beneficence. The rugged and frightening mountain or the picturesque garden are both imbued with a significance with which we can engage. We are concerned by our surroundings.

We should be more precise: once again, it is not the particular surroundings that are the point, it is the world generally. To understand anybody, you must understand his or her world, understand how they engage with it and the significance it holds. What we cannot be – it makes no sense to think of us like this – is totally *disengaged* from the world. To be totally disengaged would be to be *unconcerned*. But what could it mean to be totally disengaged from the world? It would have to mean that nothing had meaning; not in the sense that we were depressed or fed up, but in the radical sense that there would be no meaning even in principle because it is the world that gives things their particular meaning.[2] We cannot disengage from the world. It is part of what we are. To be concerned is to be connected with and interconnected within the world. Moreover, typically, we are connected and interconnected by our relationships with other people. For human beings, it is typically human relationships that form the person's world and, therefore, their field of concern (see definition below).

Human concern – a reflection of our standing as beings of this type, engaged in the world with which we are connected and within which we are interconnected.

CONSENT AND CAPACITY

Now we turn to something much more practical: issues of valid consent and mental capacity, which are both obviously relevant to dementia care. But in discussing these practical matters, we shall come back to the notion of human concern in the special sense that we have used it. It is just worth commenting that this is an unusual approach. Without wishing to upset other authors, it is generally the case that people can write whole chapters (or books) on the issues of consent and capacity without so much as a nod in the direction of 'special senses of human concern'. Of course, it is important that these laws and some of the ethical issues they raise are understood.[3] But we wish to set out these other issues to do with treatment in the context of the field of human concern. We hope this will be instructive, but readers will have to judge.

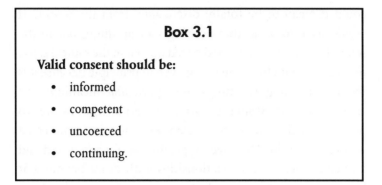

Box 3.1

Valid consent should be:

- informed
- competent
- uncoerced
- continuing.

Valid consent, in a nutshell, is summarized in Box 3.1. If you want to do anything to another adult, except in very special circumstances, you must have the person's consent and the consent must be valid. Examples of the very special circumstances would be: a police officer arresting someone for an offence, or a psychiatrist treating someone with a serious mental illness under the Mental Health Act 1983 (HMSO 1983), or a doctor in an emergency saving someone's life. In such cases, you do not need to gain consent from the person, but this emphasizes that the circumstances are extreme: crime, severe mental illness or situations of life and death. Otherwise, if you do something to someone without their consent, you can be accused of battery: it is an assault against the person. This applies to taking the person's blood pressure as much as it does to performing surgery; it also applies to undressing or making love to them.

So far, so good. It all seems very clear: no one can touch us without our permission. But now let us look at the criteria for valid consent in a little more detail (leaving 'competence' until last), especially thinking of dementia.

INFORMED

Informing someone is by no means straightforward. There are two extreme positions. In one extreme the professional (usually the doctor) knows best. This can be paternalism at its worst where no information is given, except to say that the doctor thinks the person should have the treatment. At the other extreme, the professional takes it for granted that the patient must be given all information possible without the professional expressing any real opinions. This is a consumerist approach, but it is consumerism without the shopkeeper offering any suggestions, so it is an extreme example of the view that the customer is always right. The middle way (as shown in Figure 3.1) involves judgements. In brief, it involves the patient being given information that seems relevant and helpful, but it does not involve the professional in giving excessive or burdensome information.

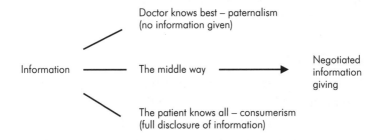

Figure 3.1 Informing: the middle way

The essence of the middle way is that there is a dynamic 'working out' or 'working through' jointly by the professional and the patient. It involves seeing how to get through or *navigate*. It involves the give-and-take of a conversation between people who are interconnected by their standing in a particular relationship (which echoes some of the themes from Chapter 2). It would be difficult to state ahead of time exactly which route should be taken. We navigate the path as we tread it. But we tread in a *concerned* way, reflecting our connectedness within the world. And this connectedness is wide: it is to the patient, his or her family, to other carers, to society, the law and to religious and moral creeds.

With this in mind, therefore, it opens up the possibility that it will be possible to convey information even if the person has moderate to severe dementia. The information may need to be conveyed slowly and it may need to be repeated, but there can be a genuine negotiation or interpretation of meaning and understanding between the professional and the person with dementia (Widdershoven and Berghmans 2006). There has to be an attitude of concern – the feeling that the person with dementia continues to share a space with us that we can understand with an appropriate approach – an attitude that takes it for granted that we remain connected to the person with dementia.

UNCOERCED

Valid consent means that the person is not coerced. If we force you to take tablets, it cannot be said that you have consented to take them. The idea of coercion is, indeed, quite repulsive to most of us. However, it is not long since outright physical restraint was relatively common in hospitals and other institutions and it still is in many parts of the world. But even in more 'advanced' nations, some forms of coercion are still routine. Chairs that people cannot get out of are, in essence, a form of restraint. It cannot then be said that the person sits all day in the chair freely. Similarly, what about when the patient is given medication secretly in food or drink? It cannot be said that the person has consented to take this medication. It is not only covert medication, but also coerced medication (Treloar, Beats and Philpot 2000). On the horizon is the prospect of electronic tagging or tracking. Electronic means of keeping someone somewhere must, again, be considered a means of restraint (Hughes and Louw 2002). There is such a thing, therefore, as covert coercion.

And yet, what if we change the word to 'cajole'? Overt coercion (ignoring covert coercion) may be repulsive, but we are not normally repulsed by the caring family who cajole their relative to attend a day centre or respite care. Encouraging someone to attend is often the lot of the family. In the context of our worldly engagement with others (reflecting our concern), encouraging or cajoling within the family seems like reasonable care. Within the residential or nursing home, the person is encouraged into the bath, despite protestations. The lines that can and cannot be crossed here are not clear cut, but reflect the messy world of morals where what is important may be the 'tone' of our dealings with people.

CONTINUING

We often overlook the fact that consent, to be valid, must be continuing. In other words, just because someone agreed to something once, it does not follow that they always agree to whatever it is. Perhaps someone has always taken her tablets without any signs of protest. Suddenly the person refuses the medication: she will not open her mouth. This, however, quickly takes us on to the key issue, which is that (in the context of dementia care) we are often not dealing with consent at all, because the person is not competent to give consent. In other circumstances, where cognitive impairment (e.g. poor memory) is not an issue, the criteria for valid consent we have already discussed are to the fore. In the case of dementia, however, the key issue is competence.

COMPETENCE OR CAPACITY

These two words can be regarded as synonymous. In the United Kingdom, 'competence' tends to be a medical term, whereas 'capacity' is a legal term. In the United States, it is the other way round. Both words refer to ability. A very important principle is that a capacity is always specific. Just because you no longer have the capacity to drive, it does not mean that you do not have the capacity to make a decision about taking an antibiotic. The other very important principle is that capacity, in legal terms, is always presumed. You cannot just presume that someone lacks a capacity; in particular, just because someone has dementia, you should not presume that he or she does not have the capacity to make decisions about finances, for instance.

Box 3.2

Principles concerning capacity:

- It is presumed.
- It is task-specific.
- It may be temporarily diminished.
- It should be facilitated.
- A decision made with capacity does not have to be reasonable or rational.

Box 3.2 shows the principles that should govern our judgements about capacity.[4] Box 3.3 provides the 'test' that someone must past in order to decide whether he or she has capacity.

Judgements about whether or not someone with dementia has a particular capacity sometimes have to be made

---

Box 3.3

The person lacks capacity if he or she:

- is unable to understand the information relevant to the decision in question
- is unable to retain the relevant information
- is unable to use or weigh that information as part of the process of making the decision
- is unable to communicate that decision.

---

formally. For example, if a serious decision is being made, such as whether or not a person should go into long-term care, it may be that a doctor will be involved in making a decision about capacity. Sometimes the decisions are so difficult (e.g. decisions about stopping treatment where this will mean that the person dies) they have to be made in a court by a judge, who will listen to the evidence of expert witnesses.

However, we should not presume that these judgements about capacity are always made by experts. Actually, they *have* to be made on a day-to-day basis. This means, therefore, that there is always the possibility that judgements about capacity can be made poorly, without enough concern. We can very easily ignore the first principle in Box 3.2 and presume that the person lacks capacity. This presumption may be true in severe dementia; but even here it would be better to presume the person does have the capacity until it is clear that he or she does not. Otherwise, the presumption that all people with dementia are 'incompetent' can quickly infect the environment and lead to a deterioration in the standing and dignity of people with dementia.[5] People with dementia are still part of the human world of concern, where their connections and interconnections are very real. As a matter of basic humanity, therefore, they deserve our respect and *care*ful treatment. But what if someone really does lack capacity? Then we should act in the person's 'best interests'.

DOING WHAT IS BEST

Judging what is best for a person is by no means easy! As we saw in Chapter 1, there are different perspectives on almost any issue. It all depends where and who you are. Our view, which seems to be that accepted in law, is that judgements about best interests must be made on a wide base. This should include taking account of the views of the person himself or herself. The person's present views should certainly be heard; but attention should also be given to the person's previous views. These might have been expressed to a member of the family or to a professional. They might even have been written down in a 'living will' or 'advance directive'. Advance directives can be very specific and, if they contain refusals of particular treatments under particular circumstances, and if the circumstances now exist, they do have a legal standing. Thus, someone might have written that if they should develop severe dementia and in the final stages of the disease start to have problems with swallowing, they would not wish to have a feeding tube inserted. This sort of *advance refusal of treatment* should be honoured.

On the other hand, the advance directive may be a statement of values, expressing the person's general beliefs and inclinations. Because a *statement of values* is not so specific, it is not easy to specify when and how it should be applied. Nonetheless, if we are concerned for other human beings, because of our mutual interconnectedness, then we should wish to take as seriously as possible the previously expressed values of the person (see Box 3.4).

Box 3.4

Determining best interests

The person making a decision about best interests must consider, so far as is reasonably ascertainable:

- the person's past and present wishes and feelings
- the beliefs and values that would be likely to influence his or her decision if he or she had capacity
- the other factors that the person would be likely to consider if he or she were able to do so.

Judging best interests, however, should go further than this. The broad base of such judgements should also incline us to talk with everyone else involved, everyone who might genuinely be able to express a view, especially concerning the views, wishes, values and inclinations of the person himself or herself. This could include not only various members of the family, but also friends (even neighbours), as well as the various professionals. Judgements about what may or may not be in the best interests of the person, therefore, must be made very broadly to reflect the views of all those genuinely concerned with the person.

To go back to our discussion at the start of this chapter, the context reflects the field of concern that surrounds a person. That is, we are inevitably engaged by and within the world by our connections and interconnections, and working out the person's best interests involves seeing, or discovering, these connections. It also involves the sort of empathic understanding – putting ourselves into the person's shoes – we discussed in Chapter 2. Understanding a person's best interests is to attempt to share his or her perspective in a field of concern. We must try to see how the person now and in the past has typically considered our world of facts and values.

REAL DECISIONS

So far we have outlined the pathway, which is built upon legal, ethical and clinical norms of practice, that has to be taken in deciding what to do for people who cannot make decisions for themselves. Let us now turn to real decisions.

Case example: controlling difficult behaviour

Graham, living with and caring for his partner of 34 years, Edward, was faced with the dilemma of whether or not to administer Edward's medication secretly when Edward refused to take it. Edward's behaviour, without the medication, could become aggressive and there had been a number of occasions when he had hit Graham. The dilemma for Graham was that Edward would become violent if he did not take the medication and Graham feared that this behaviour could possibly mean Edward having to be detained under compulsory powers (e.g. 'sectioned' under the Mental Health Act [HMSO 1983] in England and Wales), thus removing Edward from their shared home. However, Graham also believed that Edward had a right to choose whether or not to take the medication. Furthermore, Graham was also of the opinion that had Edward been well, he would have been mortified at the thought of hitting Graham, whom he loved very much. Caught between his desire not to be subject to violence, his belief that Edward had a right to choose, and the possible consequences for their life together, Graham chose to administer Edward's medication surreptitiously.

Case example: artificial feeding and hydration

One day, Akhila, a woman with dementia, stopped eating. She showed little or no interest in food and when encouraged to eat refused to open her mouth. Staff were concerned about her health and so it was suggested that artificial feeding might be considered. Akhila's daughter, Nishtha, was very much against this idea because previously when her mother had had tubes inserted into her arm Akhila had not understood what was happening, had become distressed and had tried to rip the tubes out. What was certain was that without artificial nutrition and hydration, Akhila would die. The doctor was of the opinion that Akhila's refusal to eat might only be a temporary phase and that if she could be seen through this phase, she might 'bounce back'. Nishtha, however, thought that artificial feeding would only prolong her mother's life rather than enhance its quality. Nishtha and the staff disagreed strongly and an impasse was reached.

In both of these cases we can follow the pathway pointed out previously in the chapter: we can assess the person's capacity and, if he or she does not have capacity, we can act in his or her best interests, being careful to define this broadly and base a good deal of weight on the views, if they are known, of the person concerned. We can at least try to work out what the person would have wanted under these circumstances. In a really difficult case we might have to seek the help of the court to decide what is best.

In Edward's case, it would have been entirely wrong for Graham to give him medicine secretly if Edward had the capacity to make a decision for himself. But given that this was not the case, the decision in terms of Edward's best interests was based on Graham's estimation that Edward would not have wished to behave as he was prone to do without the medication. This judgement by Graham could (in theory) be challenged, but the fact that they had been in a close and caring relationship for so many years would tend to suggest that Graham was likely to have the greatest insight into what Edward might have thought was best.

If we presume that Akhila also lacks capacity to make a decision, it is again necessary to make a judgement about her best interests. In this case, however, the views on what might be best for her differ. If there was no way of agreeing, a court order might have to be sought. One point to note is that, although it sounds as if the staff and Akhila's daughter have fallen out over their disagreement, this need not be the case. Both sides want the same thing, namely the best for Akhila. What they face together is a very difficult decision and a very important one. They need to be extremely honest with each other (in Chapter 5 we shall discuss communicative ethics, which suggests that the right decision will emerge from open and honest communication). They need to immerse themselves in the details of the case, and to share all of the history in order to understand their different perspectives. The daughter may be thinking of her mother as she once was; the staff may be thinking of other people who have done well with this sort of treatment. The daughter may have a particular view of where her mother is in her life history, which may be at odds with the view of the staff. (Thinking about narrative histories as a way of solving ethical problems is again something we discuss in Chapter 5.) They may have different views about the likely benefits or risks of treatment, which need to be shared, as well as different views about the quality of Akhila's life (another topic for Chapter 5). Discussing all of these issues carefully might lead to a shared way forward, a navigation or 'working out', requiring careful negotiation.

Case example: treating other conditions

Brian, an elderly man with dementia, was being cared for by his wife, Margaret. Subsequent to being diagnosed with dementia, Brian was also diagnosed as having lung cancer. Further investigations would be necessary to determine the extent of the cancer and the prognosis for treatment. Margaret, however, did not think that Brian would understand the necessary investigations and treatments and thought it would be cruel to put him through all of this. However, without further investigation, the prognosis was that Brian would live for only a further one to two years. With treatment, Brian might live for much longer, though his quality of life might be diminished by chemo- or radiotherapy. Margaret, in discussion with Brian's consultant, decided to take a wait-and-see approach.

When we come to Brian, the same considerations apply as applied for Edward and Akhila. However, without further information, we would have to say that the possibility that Brian might have the required capacity to make a decision needs to be taken very seriously. Perhaps in this case (we do not know) the key point is the need to recall the principle that the person's ability to participate in decisions should be facilitated (Box 3.2).

What we also wish to suggest, however, is that in (what we are calling) the messy world of morals, it may be that the real issue in these cases is our level of *concern*. We, as health and social care workers, need to be engaged with the people we look after. We are, in any case, embedded in the particular context with them and their friends and families. *The contextual details and our level of genuine concern will help us to make the correct decisions.*

This is not to deny that there will be very important facts to be considered. For instance, we need to bear in mind the potential side effects of the various treatments and the evidence that they will be worthwhile in these particular cases. We need to know, for instance, that the evidence in favour of using percutaneous endoscopic gastrostomy (PEG) tubes in dementia is not good (Finucane, Christmas and Travis 1999). Nevertheless, once we have the facts at our disposal, our position as professionals who have genuine concern will still be crucially important. This will partly be the case because the decisions will not in the end be solely made on the basis of the evidence or facts. Of equal importance will be the values that everyone brings to bear. We do not just require, therefore, evidence-based practice, but values-based practice too (Fulford 2004). Not only do we require open and honest communication about the facts of the matter, but also there will have to be open and honest discussions about the values, which may conflict.

Genuine concern and engagement will encourage empathic understanding. Crucial here, too, will be our abilities to communicate by effective listening and empathic responses. We shall need to convey factual information sensitively, whether it is to the person with dementia, or to the family and other carers. In addition, we must be able to understand and respond to the views and values of *all concerned.* Successful negotiation and navigation, based on empathic understanding, through the field of concern (which is made up of facts and values) is more likely to bring us to an outcome that is not only acceptable, but also the right outcome in the circumstances. However, being concerned and empathic does not necessarily mean simply giving way to someone else's position. We may have to take an uncomfortable stand, but if we do so it should be in the context of empathic understanding and broad negotiation and discussion. And in the end our position should reflect our concern and reflect our deep engagement with all those involved.

CONCLUSION

In this chapter we have dealt with issues that arise in connection with treating people with dementia. This will always involve considering consent and capacity and, where the person's capacity to make decisions is impaired, best interests. We then turned to consider some examples of real decisions in dementia care. This discussion has revealed:

- the importance of knowing the relevant facts about the potential outcomes of treatment, including the potential for treatments to cause harm

- the need to assess the person's capacity to consent, which should include attempts to facilitate the person's ability to contribute to decisions if at all possible

- the requirement that judgements about the person's best interests should be made, after broad and careful communication, with empathic understanding

- the extent to which this is likely to raise issues relating to the person's values and the deeply held convictions of all concerned

- the importance, therefore, of an open and honest discussion and negotiation with these values in mind.

To return to our starting point, how all of this goes will depend upon and require the sort of genuine care and concern that reflect our standing as human beings mutually engaged in our shared world.

NOTES

1. The philosopher Martin Heidegger (1889–1976) also used the notion of 'concern', but in a technical way. Nevertheless, what we are saying here is not completely foreign to his way of thinking. For a basic introduction to the work of Heidegger, see Lemay, Pitts and Gordon (1994).

2. Another giant thinker from the twentieth century, Ludwig Wittgenstein (1889–1951), had much to say about the nature of meaning. He emphasized that when we understand the meaning of a word, we understand its use. That is, we understand the context in which the word makes sense. The importance of context is something that will emerge in what we say. For a short introduction to the work of Wittgenstein, see Grayling (2001).

3. Because we do not intend to go through every aspect of consent and capacity possible, interested readers may wish to consult Department of Health (2001) or Hope *et al.* (2003) for more details on legal and ethical considerations.

4. These principles, along with the other details relating to capacity and best interests that follow, are taken from the Mental Capacity Act 2005 for England and Wales (TSO 2005), which comes into effect in 2007. Readers from other jurisdictions should seek guidance on their own legal frameworks.

5. Examples of how this happens can be found in Sabat (2001).

Chapter 4

Keeping Them Safe

INTRODUCTION

Whether or not it is true, the picture we have of (what we call) 'primitive' civilizations is that, while the men were off being hunters, the women remained at home to look after the young and old. Of course, there were not that many old people because the average lifespan was short. Things have changed. People now live much longer. One consequence of this is that there are more people with dementia because the rate of dementia goes up as people get older. Thus, about 750,000 people in the United Kingdom have dementia. This represents roughly 5 per cent of the total population aged 65 and over, and rises to 20 per cent in those over 80 years of age. It is estimated that by 2026 there will be 840,000 people with dementia in the United Kingdom.

Not everything has changed, however. Although both men and women now go out to work, it remains the case that the great burden of care largely falls on the shoulders of women, be they spouses, offspring, in-laws or even just neighbours. It is an entirely justified feminist point to indicate the inequity as regards the burden of care. Nevertheless, it should not be overlooked that a significant number of professional and informal (usually family) carers are men. Still, the point about inequity is a political one, which is worth making. We wish, alternatively, to raise another point. Perhaps there are intrinsic characteristics to care that are in some sense feminine, but which can be demonstrated by men too. More than that, we would argue that men *must* show these qualities in order to show proper care. In this chapter we shall start by looking at the notion of feminist ethics and then move on to consider the virtues. The issue we shall be considering in relation to dementia is that of safety.

FEMINIST ETHICS

In 1982, Gilligan suggested that men tend to think and talk of morality in terms of rights, autonomy and justice, whereas the female approach emphasizes caring, responsibility and interrelationships (Gilligan 1982). Later, Noddings (1984) developed a 'feminine' ethic based on the caring shown by individuals. This idea of caring was regarded as a built-in disposition. In other words, the feminine notion of caring is very like the idea of *concern* that we discussed in Chapter 3. It reflects part of what we are as human beings who occupy the same moral space – i.e. the world – in which we have to interrelate in a particular fashion, namely with care, whether we are male or female.

This 'ethic of care' is often contrasted to an 'ethic of justice' or the principlist approach that we discussed in Chapter 1. Rather than being based on universal principles or an adherence to rules, an ethic of care emphasizes the importance of relationships, the uniqueness of situations and individuals, and the necessity for good communication between people. In this ethic, reasoning *and* emotional response are important elements in the decision-making process. As such, the whole of the person is involved, not just the analytical reasoning side. The Self is defined in terms of how we relate to others (Kitwood 1997). Rather than being an automonous, independent individual, the Self is seen as related to and interdependent on others, connected through and responsive to the needs of others as they arise in the messiness of real life. Ethics is thus, in large measure, the creation, maintenance and promotion of healthy relationships. But how will these caring dispositions be worked out in particular cases?

ISSUES OF SAFETY

Let us turn to the issues of safety that may be relevant to dementia. These will, among other things, include driving, finances, the use of medication, dressing, cooking and other activities of daily living. In the case examples below we shall consider aggression, inappropriate behaviour and wandering.[1] In each case, we would suggest that a good and more acceptable outcome is achieved when the key ideas inspired by feminine ethics come into play. That is, we need an ethic of care characterized by:

- an emphasis on the importance of relationships

- an appreciation of the uniqueness of the situated individual

- a commitment to good quality communication.

Case example: aggression

Leslie had been staying in a residential home for about two months when the local authority claimed not to have the funding. His son, Paul, had paid for the bed but there was uncertainty as to what might happen and Leslie had periods of frustration because he did not really know what was going on, One day Leslie, because he was getting frustrated and angry, went up to the manager and said, 'I feel like dotting someone on the nose.' Rather than viewing this as a potentially violent situation, symptomatic of Leslie's dementia, or a problem to be resolved by medical intervention, the manager said to him, 'Leslie, that's terrible, it's not me you want to dot on the nose is it?' And Leslie, being a fairly gentlemanly individual, thought the idea that he might dot a woman on the nose was absolutely horrid. 'Oh no, no', he said. 'Of course not, no, no, absolutely not.' In reality, the manager was involved in the problem, but she was able to diffuse the situation by saying: 'Well, come and tell me what the problem is and then if someone needs dotting on the nose, we'll go and dot that person together.'

In Leslie's case the manager was able to make use of her relationship with him in order to avoid trouble. She appreciated his individual problem and was able to spend time listening to him, which is of course part of good communication. She could have tried to fob him off or dismiss his worries, but she recognized his sense of uncertainty and frustration. Things might have gone otherwise if his frustration had been allowed to build up. It would be hard to deny that this was the right thing to do.

In the following case Georgina is inevitably pulled this way and that by her relationships. Of course, she also has duties and both the possible consequences of Mark's actions and the principles of doing good, avoiding harm and respecting autonomy are relevant. But Georgina has to make a decision about what to do from where she stands in relation to her husband, their granddaughter and other children. In deciding what to do, she may well wish to think about what Mark would have wanted, but she was also able to discuss matters with other people, including professionals. The issue of safety cuts both ways: the children need to be kept safe, but so too does Mark, who may be open to prosecution or deliberate harm from others should he act inappropriately. Minimizing the risks may well involve curtailing his freedoms and communicating the risks to others. The ethic of care suggests that these measures are taken as a matter of concern from within the relationship rather than because a rule or principle dictates a particular solution.

Case example: inappropriate behaviour

Georgina was caring for her husband, Mark, who had dementia. Once, while on holiday with their daughter and granddaughter, Mark had made some very inappropriate sexual remarks about his granddaughter, remarks that concerned Georgina very much. Mark had also taken to standing in the park watching young children. Georgina was very aware of the potential danger in the situation, as she had trained as a social worker, but at the same time she did not want to have her husband labelled as a child molester or have legal proceedings instigated against him. Torn between her desire to protect her granddaughter and (possibly) other children and her loyalty to her husband, she debated how to address her concerns without involving social services or the police.

Case example: wandering

Leonard, caring for his wife, Grace, was asked how he had dealt with the problem he faced when Grace wanted to go out at unreasonable or inconvenient times:

> We have actually pretty recently solved the problem of wandering. It was a particular problem when I resisted all her demands to go out or to go home, or to do whatever she wanted to do. And I would try to reason with her, argue with her that it was not appropriate or this was her home, or whatever.
>
> Now that *always* caused *enormous* anxiety and often finished with her rushing out of the door; or the minute my back was turned she would put on her coat and go. And the way we've resolved it quite reasonably is that I now simply go along with whatever it is that she wants. So if she says, 'I want to go home', I go along quite happily with that and I tell her that I will go part of the way with her. We get the car out and we drive around, sometimes we park the car in the town, she says, 'It's now time for me to go off on my own', and we park the car. And I'd say, 'Well, I'll go a little way with you'. And then after about half an hour, three-quarters of an hour I *know* that she's coming out of that particular period of stress and anxiety and I say, 'Would you like to go home?' 'Oh yes, I think I'd like to do that.' And so we're back as it were in the real world and we come back and she's usually quite calm at that point.

Of course, it would be possible to ask whether this would be the right thing for all carers to do. The answer is that different carers manage things differently from within their relationships. As we discussed in Chapter 2, our interrelatedness is a feature of our humanity. But relationships are different. Not everyone would have been able to behave as this husband did. Whatever the chosen solution, it would need to be worked out for the individuals concerned in a given context. For instance, it might be that medication is required, with all the potential for side effects; but if this is the way to support the person continuing to live at home, it might be the right solution.

What would we say, however, within the confines of a nursing home? It is all very well, it might be argued, for a fit relative to take the person out for a walk or find some other means to calm her down, but if a strong and determined man with dementia is agitated and potentially aggressive in a care home, for instance if he were constantly trying to leave through the fire escape, it might be practically impossible to do anything other than restrain him by various means – e.g. chemically, physically or by electronic means, such as tagging. Those in charge of the home might point to the duty of care: surely we have a duty to keep people safe?

Well, this is certainly true. The example we have used and the approach of feminine ethics, however, suggest something else. Instead of thinking of duties and consequences (which might indeed be dire if the man were to escape from the home), it might be that we should also think of where the individual person stands and his perspective. This should include some consideration being given to his relationships. It is not that this is an easy option; certainly not in terms of time and commitment. On the one hand, the thought that we have a duty to keep the person with dementia safe and the fear of the consequences should he get out onto the busy street might make us reach for some calming or sedating tablets. On the other hand, the thought that the central issue is one of relationship suggests that we should strive to know the person better, so that he is understood, and we should be willing to spend more time just *being with* him, rather than *doing to* him.

Now, it remains the case that we might yet require the sedating medication. Indeed, it might be even worse: perhaps the resident can no longer be cared for appropriately in this home and will need to be transferred to a higher level of care. But the notion of relationship opens up other possibilities. Maybe, through our discussions with the family, we shall come to understand more about why he is constantly trying to leave. Maybe we shall be able to devise a strategy to meet the need that drives this behaviour (Stokes 2000). Maybe, even if we cannot, the family will be able to take him out for a walk at times. But maybe there is an activity with which he will engage within the home. Maybe we shall feel more motivated to find activities that are genuinely meaningful to him. Or maybe simply *being with* him will be enough. Maybe having a familiar face close to hand more often, speaking in a kindly way to him, will be reassuring. Maybe, even if this is not enough, it will make the process of encouraging him to take medication easier.

BEING WITH AND EMPATHY

The notion of *being with* deserves further consideration. It is central to a theme that is emerging in our discussions of how difficult decisions, which are usually ethical, are dealt with in the context of dementia care. We saw in Chapter 2 the extent to which we are located as human beings in relationships. To use Buber's phrase again, we are engaged in 'I–Thou' relationships. We are properly understood in the context of our relationships with other people. In Chapter 3, we discussed the extent to which the way we are located in a context, which is characterized by our human relationships, means that – by our nature – we are concerned or engaged with others. And now, in discussing how we keep people with dementia safe, we are pushing forward the notion of *being with*. To be with someone is to place ourselves alongside him or her. It is to acknowledge them as people with whom we engage and for whom we are concerned. *Being with* tends to be contrasted with *doing to*. We do things to other human beings in an objectifying way. They need feeding, toileting, dressing, and so on. When we just *do to* others we act in a task-directed fashion. The task is to dress her or quieten him. To focus on the task is to turn the person into an *object* of care, which reflects (to use Buber again) an 'I–It' relationship. To *be with* is to focus on the *subjective*, on how it is now for the person to be in this situation. It concerns empathy; it is to do with putting ourselves in the shoes of others; it is to understand them (i.e. empathic understanding).

The final message is that it becomes easier to accomplish tasks for someone (which is the empathic equivalent of 'doing to') once we have *been with* them. Persons with whom we have empathy, for whom we have understanding, are more likely to allow us to do things to them because there is a genuine relationship. To be someone with dementia is to be in greater need of just this sort of empathic understanding because it is, in part, by this type of understanding that our personhood is maintained. That is to say, part of what it is to be a person is to be part of a web of such human relationships. These relationships contribute to our standing as persons. In the case of people with dementia, however, where the possibility of understanding can be increasingly difficult, the need for *being with* becomes more acute, because it is by this means that a relationship (however tenuous) will be created and personhood maintained. The need for good-quality relation-ships, reflected in good-quality care, is exactly the sort of thing Kitwood (1997) was interested in when he promoted a new culture of dementia care.

PERSPECTIVISM AND MALIGNANT POSITIONING

So the notions of 'being with' and 'empathic understanding' link up. They also connect to the approach in ethics that has been called perspectivism (see definition below).

> **Perspectivism** – an ethical decision cannot be made blind to the points of view of those who have a legitimate interest in the case.

This simply means that, in trying to decide how to solve a moral dilemma, we should take seriously the different points of view of all the relevant people involved in the dilemma. Considering the different perspectives in this way forces us to be empathic, to try to stand where others stand. Too infrequently is this tried in dementia care. There has been a tendency to exclude people with dementia from important decisions. Of course, for the most part, this has been for very understandable and benign reasons. Sometimes, however, as in the case of not telling a person with dementia the diagnosis, the benign reasons may be benignly paternalistic. In other words, even if we do not think of the person as an 'It', we do have an inclination to devalue or undermine his or her standing. The American psychologist Steve Sabat refers to this as 'malignant positioning' (Sabat 2006). In other words, we place the person in a situation so that, by our attitudes, he or she cannot achieve the social or personal recognition due. Instead, the person is seen as more or less incompetent. At its worst, it is the very selfhood of the person that is undermined. So, even if the person is not an 'It', he or she may be regarded as a child. Thus, the infantilized adult requires to be kept safe, cannot be trusted to make decisions, needs constant care and supervision, and must even be talked to in a particular (i.e. patronizing) way (Cayton 2006).

Perspectivism counters these tendencies as does *being with*. Perspectivism requires us to make an intuitive, yet rational, leap: what might be the concerns of someone in this person's situation? *Being with* encourages the process by making it more likely we shall make the correct intuitive and rational leaps. One daughter, Kashka, said that the process of making decisions on behalf of her mother was a nightmare and that:

> the only thing you can do is ask yourself whether the person you're acting on behalf of would have done it that way. If the answer is yes, that helps.

Another daughter, Ingrid, said of her relationship with her mother:

> I think our relationship was close enough for me to have a fair idea – if not more so – of what my mother would have wanted. So when I made a decision for her, I probably wasn't far off making the kind of decision she would have made if it had been her choice.

PERSPECTIVISM AND THE LAW

The benefit of perspectivism is, in part, that it alerts us to the perspectives of the person with dementia. One point to note is that the person with dementia may well have had a definite opinion on what he or she would have wanted to happen under the present circumstances. These views might have been expressed by word of mouth to relatives, but they might also have been written down in the type of advance statement of values we discussed in Chapter 3. We need to recall again the various ways in which it seems proper to make decisions for people when they are unable to do so for themselves. A key principle, for instance, enshrined in the opening section of the Mental Capacity Act 2005 (TSO 2005) and recorded in Box 3.2, is that we must presume the person is competent. The notion of perspectivism hammers this point home: we need (at least) to try to involve people in decisions that affect them. So we should *try* to find out what their views (or perspectives) might be.

There is however another side to this story, because we should be trying to understand the perspectives of the carers too, be they family or formal carers. Uppermost in the minds of many carers will be the issue of safety. It is the worry over safety that creates much of the stress that surrounds caring for people with dementia. There is no sidestepping the issue. Sometimes the need to make the person safe will involve the use of compulsory detention; that is, the person's freedom will be taken away. Now the important point to see is that it cannot be just taken for granted that a person with dementia – because of the dementia – loses his or her rights.

Indeed, Article 5 of the European Convention on Human Rights states that 'Everyone has the right to liberty' (Council of Europe 2003). Nevertheless, there are a number of circumstances under which individuals can have their right to liberty taken away, for instance if they are murderers. There are circumstances when a person with dementia can be detained too, but the important point is that this does not happen on a whim! There must be good reasons and there must be a proper process for any detention to be legal.[2] Emphasizing the human right to liberty, however, should make us see how, from the perspective of the person with dementia, to be kept somewhere that is not of their choosing must be a profound affront to the person's sense of dignity.

Still, while holding this perspective in mind, the process encouraged by perspectivism entails that we should involve, insofar as it is possible, all those other people concerned with the care of the person with dementia. We emphasized the importance of this process in Chapter 3. Such an inclusive process is right and proper, but only if there is some balancing of the different views, including the views of the person with dementia. Resorting to the law in order to make such decisions, although in day-to-day decision-making is unusual, it is a sign of good care inasmuch as it makes plain the process of weighing up everyone's views; it also emphasizes the importance of such decisions. In a similar way, then, even when the law is not involved in a formal fashion, it is good practice to go through the process of taking into account the different perspectives of all concerned, especially the perspective of the person with dementia, and recording how the different views have been weighed up and balanced in the making of the eventual decision.

Case example: refusing medication

When Derek was faced with his wife refusing to take her medication he was concerned that she would deteriorate or become very ill if she did not take it. He spoke to the doctor about this and decided that his wife's wishes should be respected with regard to the anti-dementia drug. However, when it came to the medication for her chronic airway disease, he was of the opinion that his wife might be seriously ill or die if she did not take it. He consulted his doctor and other carers and finally made the decision that the best thing to do was to administer that particular medication surreptitiously.

We can, once again, consider Derek's decision from the standpoint of an ethic of care: his concern reflects his deep relationship with his wife; he takes her individual circumstances into account not only by trying to respect her wishes, but also by making a judgement about what is and is not necessary for her in her particular circumstances; and he communicates appropriately with other people involved in her care in order to make a decision. His decision was not simply the result of weighing up principles, nor was he dogmatically following a particular theory of what a good action might be. Rather, he was acting out of concern from within the context of his relationship and it would probably make more sense to him to say that he just acted instinctively, as if by intuition. To return briefly to the theme of Chapter 1, moral intuition is another way of discussing conscience. We shall now develop the theme that our instinctive actions reflect our inner dispositions and that we act well when we act in ways that allow us to become better people.

FROM FEMININE ETHICS TO THE VIRTUES

We saw at the start of the chapter how feminine ethics helped to refocus the discussion about difficult decisions. We have come back to the idea that formally or informally the legal process must be adhered to. We have come back to an emphasis on rules and rights through the discussion of perspectivism. However, we must not lose sight of the way in which perspectivism was intended to emphasize the viewpoint of the person with dementia. To return to our grand theme, the person with dementia stands in a context of relationships. Feminine ethics emphasizes our interrelationships and the notion of caring as a built-in disposition. This brings us to the concept of a virtue, where a virtue is an inner disposition that, in some sense, aims at what is good. And this allows us to talk about virtue ethics.

Virtue ethics – we know what the right action or the good decision would be if we know what the virtuous person would do.

The appeal of virtue ethics is that, whatever the processes and outcomes in our decision-making, there is another aspect to be considered. Virtue ethics suggests that, although processes and outcomes are important, our inner dispositions – the source of our actions – must also be important. If I ought to do what the virtuous person would do, I should be acting in accordance with the virtues. That is, I should show charity, truthfulness, compassion, faithfulness, generosity, prudence, and so on. If I act in accordance with these virtues, I should have acted well. This seems to make some sense. If, for instance, I try to be compassionate it seems unlikely that I would deliberately inflict pain on someone. If I try to be true, it seems unlikely that I would be deceitful. If by inclination I am prudent, then I shall try to do things in such a way as to bring about a good outcome. This virtue is also known as practical wisdom.

One thing about the virtues is that they are acquired by training and education. We learn to be honest. We appreciate from our own experience the benefits of charity. Practical wisdom also comes from experience. It allows us to see how a difficult situation might be navigated. We see a way through and we can retain a sense of balance and optimism because, based on our experience, we tend to anticipate correctly how things will go. But the virtuous person is not authoritarian and cocksure, because he or she will also have the virtues of charity and humility. This highlights, therefore, an important aspect of virtue ethics, which is that it places weight on the way in which things are done, not just on whether the person can say that they did the right thing (Hursthouse 1999).

Thus, it may well be that the right thing to do is to keep people with dementia safe. There may be no other option. Nevertheless, the way in which we do this needs to be judged. We need to take account of the other perspectives because this is to show charity and good sense. We need to listen to the concerns of others as a matter of compassion and humility. We need to approach people gently. We go through the processes, not for the sake of simple routine and not simply in order to follow a guideline, but because the process is a way of taking the values of all concerned in a serious-minded fashion. To be serious minded about something as important as a person's liberty is to show good sense and is itself a virtue. Following reasonable guidelines is also a matter of practical wisdom inasmuch as they help us to navigate our way through difficult decisions. One of the key things, according to virtue ethics, is not just the outcome, but what we *become* in doing what we do and in making the choices we make.

Peter saw caring for his wife, Carole, as having made him a better person:

> in a strange sort of way I feel I'm a better person now than I was say ten years ago. I think I'm more tolerant by and large. I'm more patient. I'm more outgoing in the sense that I realized that if Carole's to lead the best possible life then we have to be part of a community of people who are going through the same situation. I look for every oppor-tunity for social events that bring us together with other people, not just like-minded people but sometimes other things as well. Whereas I think a few years ago I was much more inclined to turn down those kinds of invitation. So I am more socially outgoing. I think I'm better now with people that I notice in the community or in groups that we belong to who clearly are suffering, who are in need, I think I'm more willing to make the first move and to try to

support them or say something which is helpful or comforting. So I think in those sorts of ways perhaps I am a rather better person than I was ten years ago: certainly less self-satisfied and self-preoccupied than I was then.

In Peter's case we see how it might be possible that caring, done in the right way, with genuine concern, can itself make us better people. We become more compassionate, for instance. It is easy to see how the virtues are essential for carers. When asked what made a good carer, Saalim replied:

> I think it is terribly important that they show love and compassion. I use these words many times but they have got to be that sort of a person, to be a caring person you must show love and compassion otherwise you can't care. To be a carer you've got to be proficient in many avenues and one of them, as I say, is love and compassion.
>
> So you've got to be a good listener, you've got to show love and compassion and you've got to know when to get help and when to leave it. And you've got to be very patient; otherwise if you're short tempered there's no point in taking the job on, because you've got to allow the patient to make the running as it were and you've got to understand why they're doing certain things and you can't do that if you're intolerant. You've got to be very tolerant and if you're not tolerant then you ought to pack it up and find something else to do.

Leonard found:

> at first that patience wasn't the best of my virtues in regards to when, what I saw as stupid things being done weren't stupid to the person who was doing them. I got quite irritated and as I got tired said things I shouldn't have said when in reality I should have tried to keep calmer. If you can do that from the beginning I think it's a

good thing but I didn't, I just, I was sort of in at the deep end and very worn out and tired and things like that. But if you can do more coaxing and keep your patience then that's a good thing, that is really a good thing. Because they don't know they're irritating you, they just think they're doing whatever they want to do I suppose. If they do want to go out and it's raining, like I said, 'No', what I should have said was, 'I'll get a brolly and we'll go', that's what I should have done. At the time I didn't. It's having a lot of patience and doing it with a good heart. Well, you must do it with a good heart because you love them I suppose.

Case example: maintaining choice

Matthew, caring for his wife, Jayne, was particularly concerned that Jayne should be able to choose what she had to eat even though she had lost all language ability and had little understanding of what it meant to choose in advance. Consequently, Matthew used to prepare three or four different dishes every evening and place them in front of his wife so that she could still choose what she would have for dinner. In so doing, Matthew was expressing his love for his wife, while simultaneously demonstrating the virtues of charity and compassion.

CONCLUSION

It is striking to see this reference to love, because it is not a concept that features much in most textbooks of moral philosophy. At the start of Chapter 3 we discussed how the notion of concern has to be understood in terms of our way of being in the world. Stephen Post, one of the leading thinkers on ethical issues in dementia (see Post 2000), makes a link

between 'our universal human needs' and the requirement for
love, which he points out is how Kitwood (1997) defined the
main psychological need of people with dementia.

> Persons with cognitive disabilities need the emotional
> sense of safety and joy, *and seem to reveal in the clearest way our*
> *universal human needs.* The first principle of care for such
> persons is to reveal to them their value by providing atten-
> tion and tenderness in love. (Post 2006, p.232 [emphasis
> in original])

In this chapter we have:

- considered how a feminine ethic of care
  emphasizes the importance of relationships, the
  uniquely situated nature of individuals, and the
  need for good-quality communication

- discussed how empathic relationships are likely to
  be encouraged by the notion of *being with*

- shown how taking the unique perspective of
  individuals can help to avoid placing the person
  with dementia in a disadvantaged position while,
  at the same time, encouraging a broadly based
  process of estimating what might be right in the
  difficult circumstances of having to provide people
  with safety

- finally, come back to the idea that our decisions,
  in order to be ethical, must reflect our inner
  dispositions, which must in turn be in keeping
  with the virtues if we are to become good carers.

Being virtuous requires us to engage in a genuine way with those we care for, as a matter of compassion and charity, and this entails a concern that amounts to love. As Post suggests, this is nothing other than a non-negotiable part of our 'common humanity':

> The person with dementia...is part of our common humanity as an emotional and relational being and therefore must be treated with care and respect. Only a view of humanity that excludes emotion and relationality would ignore this and such a view would be both callous and inhumane. (Post 2006, pp.232–233)

NOTES

1. These three expressions – aggression, inappropriate behaviour and wandering – are commonly used in connection with people with dementia. However, they raise some important issues. In each case the behaviour is regarded as 'inappropriate', but from the perspective of the person with dementia the behaviours may not be inappropriate at all. The 'aggression' may be justified self-defence; the behaviour (which is also sometimes called 'challenging') may only be inappropriate or challenging to others but might make perfect sense to the person with dementia; similarly, the 'wandering' may reflect a perfectly reasonable desire to go somewhere to achieve something. Our use of the terms is not intended to encourage the view that the person's behaviour cannot be understood; our clinical and ethical stance is that we should try to understand these behaviours, which may mean that our commonly used language should change.

2. We are not entering into the difficult area of mental health law, but practitioners need to be aware of the relevant laws and legal frameworks and guidelines that govern where they work.

Chapter 5

It's the Quality that Counts, but How do We Decide?

INTRODUCTION

'Quality of life' is a phrase that trips easily off the tongue. It is easy to accept the argument that it is this – quality of life – that makes the difference. Who would wish to live a long but miserable existence? This is not just true for people with dementia, it is true for us all. If our lives lack quality, we feel impoverished: we are literally poorer if we have nothing of quality in our lives. In healthcare this has led to the slogan 'life to years, not years to life'. In our research with family carers of people with dementia, the notion of quality most often reared its head in connection with the idea of life being extended or preserved.

For example, Ruth (who cared for her husband) talked about balancing quality of life with the possible benefits of artificial feeding:

> There is another way in which I think there may be something up ahead. My husband's starting to have problems

with swallowing now, and up ahead I think there may be the question of 'Do we artificially feed him?' and I think my answer to that is 'No'. All along I've been led by the maxim that the quality of life is more important than the length of life. And again I'm making the decision on my husband's behalf and the weight of that is enormous.

Another carer, Louise, was faced with the decision of whether she should subject her husband to treatment for lung cancer, when he might not understand the treatments and become distressed by them:

> But the consultant said rather than keep dragging my husband back for appointments he would look at putting the palliative care on to the GP [general practitioner] in the long term. So I said, 'Well you know I just feel that his quality of life is more important than prolonging it.' And the consultant said he was glad I'd made that decision because that was his own decision. He felt that there was nothing that he could offer that would be comfortable for [my husband] and would have any definite long-term gain.

It was usually when there was a suggestion that life could be extended that carers pointed to the quality (or lack of quality) of life. But, of course, quality of life is not simply a concept to be used to discuss when a person might die. It is all about living, so even when the question of dying has not raised its head, quality should be on the agenda. The overall aim of care, after all, should usually be to support and, if possible, improve the person's quality of life.

In this chapter we shall start by considering in a little more detail what quality of life might mean. This will lead us to consider how it can be assessed. Our conclusion will be that the notion of quality of life makes sense only if it is truly person-centred. One important aspect of person-centred care is good-quality communication. Discourse ethics captures the sense that difficult decisions require good communication. A related approach to ethical decision-making is narrative ethics, which can be a useful way to think of the very end-of-life decisions that sometimes raise a concern with quality of life for family carers. Of course, one of the reasons quality of life rears its head in connection with dementia is that we presume quality of life at the end is so poor. One question should lurk in our minds, therefore, as we discuss these issues: ought we to accept this state of affairs? This would not necessarily be an argument for extending the person's life, but it would be an argument for good-quality palliative care in dementia.

WHAT IS QUALITY OF LIFE?

In a sense we all know what 'quality of life' means. It means having a certain fitness, both mental and physical, so that we can enjoy our relationships and our surroundings. It means the potential to participate in our communities, both through worthwhile employment and by our enjoyable hobbies. At another level it means having the opportunity to appreciate cultural and aesthetic experiences. There again, quality does not solely imply being active, it might also suggest some sort of spiritual peace.

The trouble is, however, all of this is arguable. It is not necessarily that people would disagree with individual aspects in the preceding sketch of what quality of life means, but different people might wish to put different weight on different aspects. And, actually, some people might disagree with the sketch. For instance, do you really have to be physically fit to enjoy a good quality of life? (Or do you really have to have hobbies?) Are we going to say that everyone with a disability has a poorer quality of life than people without disabilities? What of people with mild or even moderate dementia? Perhaps they can experience enjoyment from relationships, from participating in social functions, from helping, or from being quiet and still in an art gallery or a church.

This can be called the *problem of domains*. What are the areas or domains of life that go to make up quality of life? Having sketched the domains, which items should be included in a particular domain? There have been numerous attempts to pin down the domains of quality of life. Not surprisingly, however, different researchers have come up with different domains and different weightings. The World Health Organization has come up with a questionnaire containing 100 items split into six domains, which has been used to compare, for instance, quality of life in dementia with quality of life in cancer (Struttmann *et al.* 1999). Other questionnaires use different questions with different domains, albeit with an overlap. Hence, quality of life is 'a confusing and complex concept' and, it has been suggested, definitions of quality of life should be left: 'to individual actors functioning with agency in their own time and space' (Bond and Corner 2004, p.109).

Why is this of significance for people with dementia? Well, if researchers cannot agree about what constitutes quality of life, we should regard their judgements about the quality of life for people with dementia sceptically. This is made even truer by another problem for those who discuss quality of life: the *subjective-objective problem*. As soon as we think about quality of life we come up against the problem that there are two aspects to it. First, there are the outer aspects, the objective factors of quality of life. If a person with dementia is incontinent of faeces, it would seem reasonable to say that this was an objective sign of low quality of life, because not being able to care for yourself in this basic way must be a matter of regret: no one would wish to be faecally incontinent. But, second, there is a subjective, more personal or inner aspect to quality of life. This depends on how the person actually feels, whatever the outer circumstances. Thus, people confined to wheelchairs commonly assert that their quality of life is good: subjectively they feel fulfilled, happy and hopeful.

To a degree this takes us back to the problem of domains: how much weight do we put on the subjective aspects and how much on the objective aspects of quality of life? In dementia, however, as communication becomes more and more difficult, the subjective aspect becomes increasingly inaccessible or hidden. We just do not know, in the end, how the person feels. So there is a great danger that we might make the wrong judgement when we are faced by difficult decisions. To return to the issue of faecal incontinence, we would probably all agree that objectively speaking this is a bad thing from the point of view of quality of life. Hence, if we see someone with severe dementia, who is unable to communicate and is faecally incontinent, we might reasonably reach the conclusion that the person's quality of life is poor. This conclusion might then influence important decisions about withholding or withdrawing treatment; that is, life-or-death decisions.

Now, the decision to withhold treatment might be quite right, and we are certainly not going to argue that faecal incontinence is pleasant for anyone. However, there may be the world of difference, from the point of view of how it is subjectively for the person, if the incontinence is managed well or poorly. The person may be washed and cleaned gently, with compassion and attention to dignity, or dealt with in an abrupt and careless fashion. Subjectively, the person may feel surrounded by love or by loathing and knowing how it is should make a difference to our estimations concerning quality of life. The ethical point is this: a decision to withhold a particular treatment (say, artificial feeding) may be morally appropriate, but the grounds for that decision may be morally inappropriate if they are based on a faulty judgement about quality of life. Moreover, if the judgement that the quality of life is poor is in fact correct, but if it is correct because the quality of care is poor, then it is exceedingly worrying that a person might be denied treatment because they are receiving poor care in the first place!

MEASURING PEOPLE

For some very good reasons researchers are often interested in measuring quality of life in people with dementia. For instance, it may be useful to try to judge whether a particular medication improves or worsens the person's quality of life. In addition, there are ethical arguments about how resources are used. Money spent on anti-dementia drugs, for example, cannot be spent on the repair of hip fractures. In order to try to be fair, health economists have developed Quality-Adjusted Life Years (QALYs) to make judgements between different types of treatment (see Hope *et al.* 2003, pp.177–183).

Despite the good reasons for measuring quality of life, however, any attempt to do so runs up against the sort of problems referred to above, namely the problem of domains and the subjective-objective problem. These problems reflect an underlying difficulty in this field, which is that we are trying to measure *qualities*, whereas we normally measure *quantities*. Furthermore, our thoughts about quality of life quickly reveal that this is a concept that will be highly individual. Of course we can make some general statements, but we soon find ourselves considering the differences between people. The solutions to the problems associated with quality of life are to think from the perspective of the person or persons concerned (that is, to be person-centred) and to think broadly (which means recognizing the innumerable ways in which people are different as persons).

Being person-centred means the problem of domains is the problem of determining the domains for this particular person, not for everyone. We can do this by finding out more about individual people: all about their history, their families and background, their likes and dislikes. The subjective-objective problem is solved by thinking broadly about the individual. Again, finding out about him or her from the family will help, but careful observation will also be important. Even when the person cannot speak there will be other bits of information, from those around or from gestures and what we might call emotional tone (the sense of happiness or unhappiness, irritability or placidity, that the person gives out), which will allow judgements to be made about the person's quality of life.

One carer, Emily, explained her change of thinking about quality of life over the period she had been caring for her husband in this way:

> if you'd said to me ten years ago at the beginning of this illness, in ten years' time my husband will become immobile, speechless, doubly incontinent, unable to do anything for himself, and really has only got his music and nourishment and human touch as the three pleasures. He's also practically blind as well… And if somebody said to me, 'Does somebody in that state have any quality of life?' I think ten years ago I'd have said, 'No'. But working with him now, caring for him now, there is still quality of life there, there are still things that he appreciates. He likes the

feel of the sun on his hands, he likes to see what he probably distinguishes as bright colours, but what they are he has no idea. He likes his music, he likes to be sung to, he likes to be played with in a way that you play with a small child and he loves human contact and cuddles and tickles and all these sorts of things. And yes, there is still a quality of life there.

In this chapter we started with a discussion of quality of life and moved to a very general point about difficult ethical decisions that might involve estimates of quality of life. People with dementia must be judged as individuals. Decisions about quality of life must be made from the perspective of the person and on the basis of a very broad assessment of what might be pertinent, recognizing the extent to which we are situated as persons in all sorts of broadening fields.

In Chapter 4 we talked of the situated individual. Now we can see why the person's being situated requires us to engage in broad consultation and assessments. We stand (or are situated) as persons of a certain physical shape and form, with certain mental strengths and weaknesses, within the context of family, society, culture and history, with particular traditions, with legal and moral codes and certain spiritual or religious views. Quality of life is particular to this standing or situatedness (Hughes 2003). Hence, there should be no off-the-shelf measuring sticks for quality of life.

This is not to say, however, that judgements about quality of life cannot be made. The families that make the judgement that the person's quality of life is too poor to warrant treatment usually do so from within a shared perspective. They are similarly situated or (to use a more colloquial expression) they know where the person concerned must be coming from. While it is all too easy to devise an inadequate measure of quality of life, there are also very sophisticated tools, which (for instance) start by assessing what the person himself or herself regards as important in order to use domains that are individual to the person. In connection with advance directives in Chapter 3, we discussed how a statement of values (which is also sometimes called a 'values history') can be useful when it comes to making decisions on behalf of someone. We also saw how values are as important as facts in the process of deciding someone's best interests.

It is also worth mentioning Tom Kitwood's novel idea of Dementia Care Mapping (DCM). This is primarily an observational tool to chart the quality of care being given to a person with dementia or within a home. However, it is a short step from quality of care to quality of life. Indeed, DCM produces a well-being score, where well-being can easily be conceived as an important component of quality of life. DCM demonstrates both of the important features necessary to arrive at a meaningful statement about a person's quality of life. First, Kitwood (1997) recognized the importance of viewing things in detail and broadly. We need to consider the day-to-day interactions of caregivers and people with dementia. Second, the judgements that need to be made should be made from the perspective of the person with dementia.

The notion of quality of life, therefore, should lead us to consider in detail what it is to provide person-centred care, where what it is to be a person is also considered broadly in terms of a multilayered situatedness (Hughes 2001). And person-centred care, therefore, involves attention to all of the biological, psychological, social and spiritual aspects of care (Brooker 2004). This form of holism – taking the full person into account – is as central to person-centred care as it is to palliative care, to which we shall return. The key aspect of person-centred care is the importance of communication in all its forms. This leads us on, therefore, to consider the relevance of discourse ethics. We started the chapter acknowledging the importance of the quality of life, but we have seen that in reality, when faced by difficult decisions, we have to turn again to the themes that have reared their heads throughout the book: the importance of context, of relationships and of empathic understanding. To these we now add the need to look in detail at the quality of care as shown by day-to-day interactions, and the importance of situated personhood. The final two approaches to ethics incorporate many of these themes.

DISCOURSE ETHICS

The idea behind discourse or 'communicative' ethics (see definition below) is that discourse itself must be respectful if the right decision is to be made.

> **Discourse (communicative) ethics** – appropriate decisions depend on an ethical base of shared, respectful discourse.

Moody put it this way:

> According to this perspective, finding the 'correct answer' to an ethical dilemma may be less a matter of agreeing on an abstract set of principles than it is a matter of sharing a commitment to free and open communication and working on behalf of institutional structures that support such communication. (Moody 1992, p. 38)

The thought is that many dilemmas result, or are made more difficult, by the inability of those concerned to face matters squarely and truthfully. This often has deep historical roots. Older people, for instance, have gradually been placed in a position, reflecting societal and political pressures, where they have no real choice. They may have to accept long-term care because there is no political will to provide alternatives. This truth can easily be glossed over; whereas, the more it is seen clearly, the more it becomes possible to consider ways to put it right. Moody's quote talks of institutional structures.

Case example: institutional loss of liberty

One man, Pietr, prior to being admitted to a residential home, enjoyed walking and he had taken a walk every day for the past 20 years. Upon admission, however, he was not allowed to go out walking without first being assessed because the staff feared that he might get lost or come to some harm, although he had never done so in the past. Because there were not enough staff available to accompany him, the rules of the home precluded Pietr from continuing his daily habit.

Here we see an institutional rule, a lack of staff, and doubt-less a worry about litigation all conspiring to prevent true person-centred care that might enhance the man's quality of life. The possibility of this occurring should have been discussed prior to admission. It may have been that facing the issue honestly (by naming it) might have led to a resolution in favour of the man being allowed to take more exercise. At a personal level, clear communication allows compromise and a more acceptable solution than if solutions are one-sided and foisted upon people.

Clinical experience shows that good-quality and truthful communication is often the way to avoid complaints when difficult decisions have to be made. Moody (1992) sugg-ests that communication should have primacy. This will often involve careful negotiation within families, or between families and professional caregivers. At the basis of much of this sort of negotiation should be an acknowledgement, according to Moody, of moral ambiguity. In other words, it can be difficult to know what is right or wrong. For instance, at what point does it become right to take over from someone with dementia? At some stage the person may need a hand with washing, but perhaps not yet.

Daniel, caring for his wife at home, reported how he had initially taken over more than perhaps he should have:

> My wife was a very, very efficient household manager but that has virtually gone although occasionally she shows a willingness and indeed an ability to do certain things like ironing although she usually leaves the iron on afterwards, or simply walks away from it in the middle and gets on with something else. She can't cook but she can help with cooking so what I normally do is suggest that she cut up the vegetables or sets the table or something like that. She doesn't do any cleaning although again from time to time she will polish a table or put a duster round but in a rather disorganized way. Initially when I seemed to be taking over responsibilities in the house she was resistant and said, 'You're taking everything away from me.' But now she's quite happy about that, she's perfectly happy for me to take the lead in the house and also in matters like shopping and so on.

NARRATIVE ETHICS

While discourse ethics stresses interrelatedness and the need for clear open communication, narrative ethics emphasizes our situatedness in interconnecting stories (see definition on p.106). It is easy enough to understand how our lives can be thought of as stories, but the implications of this way of thinking are profound. It partly implies that we create our lives: we tell our own stories. In other words, we can make things happen or not happen in our narratives. This should remind us of virtue ethics (discussed in Chapter 4), which stresses the importance of what we become by what we do. So, as professionals, we become this or that sort of person by the way we pursue our work. But, also, we step into other people's stories when we become involved with them as professionals. It is not just that we create our own stories, but we co-create the stories of others; and our own lives are co-created too (Baldwin 2005).

> **Narrative ethics** – the right decision will emerge from a correct understanding of the person's story and where they are situated in this co-created history.

One implication, therefore, of narrative ethics is that we are agents or actors in multiple interconnecting stories and we shall become something (more or less virtuous or more or less vicious) by the parts we play, by the choices and decisions we make. A second implication is that we should recognize the extent to which those we engage with are also involved in the stories of other people. The often crucial role of the family, for instance, is emphasized in narrative ethics. Finally, this way of thinking about ethics should imply that judging whether something is right or wrong for a particular person will require an appreciation of this person's particular story. And the greater the understanding the better.

As one carer, Ethan, said:

> And the quality that you have to have is to be able to step back and put aside your own frustrations and put yourself in the position of the person who is struggling with something, and just go along with them. Go along with them until they come out of it or until they access the informa-

tion that they need in such a way that they can receive it so that they can process whatever problem they've got and come out of it. And the carer needs to be able to understand the person really well so that they can understand the triggers that are going to create stability and security.

Another man, Dominic, caring for his wife, was very concerned that his actions should not cause further problems for his wife, as she might experience his actions as being 'out of synch' with how she remembered him during their married life. For example, there were times when his wife would become resistant or aggressive when Dominic was attempting to tend to her personal hygiene. Forcing her to do something against her will was not something that Dominic would normally have done as a husband:

> That, I found, a difficult situation to be in. How far do I force the issue to do what I knew had to be done without causing my wife concern, distress and causing a problem between us? That I found difficult to handle, because of the closeness because of the way we knew each other. If she understood, which I'm not sure she understood at that time. But, if she understood, she would also experience a change in me because under normal circumstances, as I just said, I would not have forced my wife to do anything in the past. If she had wanted to do it, we would have discussed it and we would have agreed whether we were going to do it or whether we're not.

For Dominic, their mutual understanding of their relationship throughout the course of their married life was key to the care he wished to provide for his wife:

> I think basically it's because my feeling for my wife and the relationship that we'd had, a historical understanding of my wife, certainly her understanding of me throughout

our married life, I didn't want her to experience any changes, any drastic changes in my attitude or behaviour. I never wanted her to experience that.

NARRATIVES AND END-OF-LIFE

Narrative ethics provides a way to approach some of the classic ethical dilemmas that arise towards the end of the person's life. (For a fuller treatment of some of the end-of-life issues raised here, see Hughes 2005 and Baldwin 2006.) For instance, if a person with dementia develops a fever, a question sometimes arises concerning to what extent this should be investigated and treated. The treatment options range from tepid sponging, using fans and paracetamol to keep the fever at bay, to intensive care with ventilation and intravenous antibiotics. It is typically at this point that many people would tend to point towards the poor quality of life of a person with dementia and say this should mean that intensive efforts to keep the person alive should not be pursued.

Winifred, caring for her husband, explained how she had made her decision not to have her husband treated:

> One of the things that I've thought about a lot recently is that when [my husband] died he had a treatable illness. If he hadn't had dementia he would have been taken into hospital and he would have been treated aggressively with antibiotics, he would have had a long convalescence and he would almost certainly have recovered from the illness. And his family and I, because I didn't make the decision, we made it jointly as a family, we decided not to treat the illness because my husband had very little quality of life left then. He wouldn't have been able to understand the treatment but he would have had to have gone into a different hospital, lots of strangers around him, lots of

invasive procedures, you could never have explained that he had to rest. We couldn't see how my husband could have got through any of that with any quality of life left at all.

Such judgements may or may not be correct, but (given the problems with the concept of quality of life) narrative ethics would suggest we should be inclined to take a broader view. We concluded our discussion of quality of life by emphasizing the importance of context, of relationships and of empathic understanding. In addition, there was the need to look at day-to-day interactions and the importance of situated personhood. These features are part of the broader view narrative ethics would commend. Context can be taken to refer to where the person is within his or her narrative. Moreover, the details of the fever – its cause, severity and the likely prognosis – will make a difference. In short, the decision about what might be right or wrong in this situation must depend on the details of the case, on an understanding of this particular person's history. And narrative ethics encourages us to consider matters both from the point of view of the person himself or herself and (as in the case above) from the perspective of the co-creators of the narrative: the family, friends and others involved in the person's care.

Furthermore, narrative suggests a place for considering the person's life as a whole. This becomes relevant, as a further example of end-of-life decision-making, in decisions about artificial nutrition and hydration. (This and other end-of-life issues are further discussed in Hughes and Louw 2005.) Nowadays there are a number of ways to keep people fed and watered, from subcutaneous drips and nasogastric (NG) tubes to percutaneous endoscopic gastrostomy (PEG) feeding. There is evidence that the use of PEG and other artificial means of feeding may not be effective. This in itself would count ethically against the use of such invasive measures (Gillick 2000). But, it can also be argued, the ethical basis for avoiding such means of feeding in severe dementia is to be found in an awareness of the person's narrative or story. Intensive care of various forms might seem wholly appropriate in other circumstances where, for instance, the chances of a cure or rehabilitation are very real. When a person has had dementia for a number of years, however, when he or she is totally dependent on others for all forms of basic care, invasive treatments might well seem inappropriate. This is decidedly *not* solely because the person has dementia (for we would not suggest the same attitude for people with less severe dementia), nor is it to do with the person's *age* (for we might suggest much the same for the younger person in this stage of dementia), but it is to do with where they are in the course of their life history. To use slightly different language, we might argue that we would tend, under these circumstances, to think that we should do the *ordinary* things, such as tepid sponging etc. for the fever and careful (e.g. slow and semi-solid) oral feeding for the person who is having difficulty swallowing, but not the *extraordinary*, such as intensive care or PEG feeding.

> **Ordinary and extraordinary means** – we are not morally bound to take extraordinary means to prolong life where this involves a disproportion between the treatment and its results, either because it would be ineffective or because it would be burdensome.

The doctrine of ordinary and extraordinary means involves an assessment of how burdensome an investigation or treatment might be for a particular person in proportion to the likely benefits. Therefore, it involves a judgement about quality of life; but it is focused on a particular person in specific circumstances (where context, relationships and attempts at empathic understanding are vital) and, moreover, it emphasizes the likely *burden* of the investigations or treatments proposed for this individual. That is, the judgement requires some sort of narrative perspective. What would this treatment mean for this person now? Any judgement about the meaning now must take into account the history that leads up to and explains how the person might feel.

The issue of artificial nutrition and hydration usually arises because of worries about swallowing. In the severer stages of dementia, control of swallowing can become impaired and the person is more likely to aspirate (i.e. food may go into the lungs) and suffer a chest infection. In the end, aspiration pneumonia can be the cause of death for many people with dementia. It often combines with a general increasing frailty, with immobility and weight loss. Under these circumstances the use of PEG feeding, for instance, may well seem burdensome given that the outcome is likely to be no better than if it were not used. Moreover, many people would wish to point to the place of feeding in the person's life.

Jennifer, caring for her mother, explained the difficulty:

> They didn't stop feeding my mother, but she chose not to eat. My father was interested in whether they ought to do a naso-gastric feed. The difficulty with that is, having started it, at what point do you decide to stop? And we felt that, knowing the person my mother was, she would have absolutely loathed the idea that you just feed somebody through the nose for the sake of an extra whatever number of days or weeks.

Similarly Rachel said:

> I think once you start getting towards tube-feeding and intravenous feeding, then for me, personally, you're going too far towards the invasive procedures that don't actually improve quality of life.

Being fed brings personal attention and care and may, for this reason, be of value to the person with dementia. Hence, many would wish to opt for conservative methods of feeding, using good positioning, with small amounts of food of the correct consistency. The aim would be to minimize the chances of aspiration while still keeping the possibility of a beneficial type of human interaction open. The narrative suggested by such an approach is quite different to the narrative of the person whose swallowing is probably temporarily impaired by a stroke, where the prospects of rehabilitation and a reasonably good recovery are highly likely. The difference in terms of treatment, between the person with end-stage dementia and the person with a stroke, involves a judgement about quality of life, *but with respect to this particular person in these singular circumstances* where possible interventions and treatments – and especially their burdens – are judged accordingly.

CONCLUSION

This chapter has concentrated on quality of life and end of life. The two notions seem to go together, but – as we said – the desire for a good quality of life is not something restricted to the end of life. It should be the aim of our care and treatment of patients. Our further discussions have led us to these thoughts:

- Our concern is with unique persons, broadly understood, where the quality of a person's life has to be understood individually.

- The multilayered context in which persons are situated argues in favour of taking a very broad view both of what might improve the person's quality of life and when balancing quality of life against length of life.

- Honest communication, as commended by discourse ethics, will help to focus on the needs of individuals over and against the requirements or routines of institutions.

- A narrative approach will also bring into view the broader aspects of a person's life, including the actors who co-create their stories, which will help when difficult decisions have to be made.

- These decisions must consider not only facts (about the effectiveness and side effects of treatments), but also the values of those most concerned.

If quality of life ought to make us focus on individual situated agents – that is, persons located in a particular context – the end of life ought to do so more forcefully. The need for good quality end-of-life care is becoming more and more apparent. The more we think of people with dementia as persons, the more it appears that palliative care – with its emphasis on physical, psychological, social and spiritual well-being – is an entirely appropriate paradigm for dementia care (Hughes, Robinson and Volicer 2005). As Post has stated:

A new form of hospice for patients with advanced [Alzheimer's disease] would revolve around the concept of 'being with' rather than 'doing to' patients beyond moderate [Alzheimer's disease], even if they have some years to live. Obviously, palliative medications and care for conditions such as skin sores would be imperative. Efforts to enhance emotional, relational, and esthetic well-being would, under such a plan, be enhanced in ways that involve family members, providing them with a sense of meaning and purpose. Through music, movement therapy, relaxation, and touch, such efforts support patients' remaining capacities. (Post 2000, p.107)

Chapter 6

Making Decisions in Practice

INTRODUCTION AND REVIEW

The unique ethical dimension to dementia care is that people with dementia, who were once able, cannot now make decisions for themselves. In Chapter 3, we indicated the correct process for making decisions under these circumstances. Such decision-making needs to accord with the local legal framework, which in the United Kingdom involves an assessment of capacity and then, if the person is not competent to make the required decision, an assessment of best interests. Ethically speaking, this legal process is underpinned by a commitment to the person: his or her ability to participate in decisions must be facilitated, past and present wishes must be given great weight and consultations should be broad, reflecting the broad basis of personhood. The philosophical basis for this ethical and legal process is that we are persons situated in contexts that are typically multilayered (Hughes 2001).

Elsewhere in the book we have stressed the importance of relationships, of good-quality communication, of taking the broad view of the person, of *being with*, of taking account of

Table 6.1 Moral theories, approaches and themes		
Moral theory	**Approach**	**Theme**
Consequentialism	Discourse (communicative) ethics	Being with
Deontology		Communication
Principlism	Feminist (care) ethics	Concern
Virtue ethics		Conscience
	Narrative ethics	Empathic understanding
	Perspectivism	Relationships
		Situated personhood

the various perspectives and the need for empathy. We have also highlighted how certain moral theories or approaches can be useful. We have considered feminist or care ethics, virtue ethics, perspectivism, discourse or communicative ethics and narrative ethics (see Table 6.1). The point about these different approaches is that they provide ways of seeing the person with dementia with his or her unique point of view as central, but they do not ignore the context of the person and the way in which the person is located in a nexus of relationships, including those with professional carers. In order to make the right decisions for people with dementia we need to engage with them. As dementia progresses this becomes more difficult unless a broader view of the person is adopted, which will enable us to come to know the person through others and through their embedding history.

In Chapter 1, we were rather dismissive of ethical theories, such as consequentialism, deontology or principlism. Of course, as we saw, these theories *can* be helpful. The crucial factor that they lack, however, is an emphasis on the essential nature of relationship. They are theories that can be applied from the outside, as it were, from an entirely objective standpoint; whereas the approaches we have commended take it for granted that decision-makers will be engaged with the situation and context surrounding the person whom the decision concerns. For this reason, in our view, these latter types of moral theory or approach are more appropriate when thinking about dementia care.

This is perhaps not so obviously true of virtue ethics. Virtue ethics, a major ethical theory with roots going back to Aristotle, stands as the alternative to consequentialist or deontological theories. It could be argued that a decision to do what the virtuous person would do, which is what virtue ethics requires, could be made from the outside, without the decision-maker having to engage with the person with dementia and his or her context. However, first, the virtuous person (*because* he or she is virtuous) is unlikely to stay disengaged and would normally wish to be aware of the perspective (in all its richness) of the person with dementia. Second, we emphasized that virtue ethics stresses what we *become* by our decisions. All this is a direct way of pulling us into the context: we are not able to make disengaged decisions because our very decisions have the potential to change us for better or for worse.

Furthermore, in Chapter 1 we stressed the extent to which ethical decisions are everywhere. Subsequently we have discussed a number of the big decisions, to do with, for example, keeping people safe and the end of life, but we should recall that there is a 'micro-ethical' decision attached to whether or not we speak to the person with dementia whom we pass in the corridor (Komesaroff 1995). There is an ethical dimension to *how* we do things as well: how we wash them, dress them, feed them and whether we do this with care and concern, or in a disengaged, callous way. One of the merits of virtue ethics is that it takes these things seriously as moral matters: the virtuous person will not ignore the humanity of people with dementia. This may not mean that the virtuous person will say 'hello' to everyone all the time! But just as it is rude or unthinking (suggesting a failure to exercise the virtue of charity) to pass someone in a corridor whom you know well without acknowledging them, so too in the case of people with dementia. The virtuous person will sometimes need to be quick in performing his or her tasks, but this would be no excuse for doing the job poorly (for example, leaving the person with dementia dirty or hungry) or doing it brutally (for example, by causing discomfort or choking).

The other theme of Chapter 1 was that the moral world is messy. We used the word 'eclectic' to describe how moral decisions are made and we focused on the matter of conscience. In this final chapter we wish to return to these ideas. Having presented a variety of approaches (and there are others!),[1] and not forgetting the major ethical theories with which we began, the question can still be asked: how do we decide what to do? Are we at liberty to pick and choose from these approaches and views (as it were) at random? In this chapter we hope to pull together these different approaches and theories by describing how decisions are actually made.

WELL, HOW DOES IT FEEL?

Our approach to ethics and moral philosophy is from practice (Dickenson and Fulford 2000). In other words, although we have thought about moral dilemmas in a theoretical way, we have also encountered them in the stories of family carers and in the hurly-burly of clinical practice. People interested in these issues sometimes wonder how practice contributes to theory. It is easy enough to see how a moral theory might be carried into clinical practice (for example, if we wish to know what the right thing to do is, we might consider a moral theory), but is the direction of travel ever reversed? We are in agreement with those who think it is (Fulford 1991). One way in which there might be traffic from practice back to theory, we would suggest, is to be found by asking how it *feels* to make ethical decisions in practice.

It is instructive to see the extent to which this question might seem to be irrelevant. A philosopher in an ivory tower (if such a person exists) might prefer to argue that how a person feels when making a decision in response to an ethical dilemma is neither here nor there. Say the person is making a really evil decision on the basis of illegitimate premises and illogical reasoning, would it matter that he or she *felt* good about it? Or, say we feel terrible about a decision, but it is the only right decision in difficult circumstances? We may have a psychological interest in these feelings, but people's actions are surely judged by criteria that include rationality, coherence and validity, rather than by how they feel.

All of this is to miss our point. Another way to misunderstand us would be to think we were suggesting anything like an emotive theory of ethics, according to which when we say something is good, all we mean is that we tend to approve of it. Our claim is certainly not that feelings determine whether something is right or wrong.

No, we are interested in something else, which is that ethical decisions are often made without any overt awareness that the decision is ethically problematic. This feeling is sometimes quite puzzling. In part this point simply restates our cry that ethics is everywhere. It is not surprising that we acknowledge the person with dementia in the corridor with a smile or word and yet do not actually note that in deciding to do this we were taking a moral step. We just do these sorts of thing (or perhaps we do not!). On reflection we might accept that there is an ethical aspect to acknowledging a person, but at the time we do not tend to think that saying 'hello' is a moral action – it is just part of normal behaviour.

The puzzling thing is when the decision is clearly ethical – for example, whether to give antibiotics to the person with severe dementia who now has a fever – and yet we do *not* feel it to be an ethical dilemma. Subjectively, it simply seems a matter of making a practical decision, which we just have to get on with. Junior doctors, for instance, sometimes note that they have spent a good deal of time at medical school discussing ethical dilemmas and then, in practice, when the decisions come along – for example, to do with withdrawing medication in the knowledge that the person will die – they often seem to be decided without long ethical debate, but just as if they were purely practical matters.

One carer put it quite explicitly in talking about the difficulty in getting his wife to take her medication:

> We went through a long session when my wife didn't want to take her medication. At the hospital they said, 'She won't take her tablets.' I said, 'Well, put them in her pudding or put them on the end of a banana.' 'We can't, the Mental Health Act says you mustn't force people to do things they don't want to.' …I wrote to the psychiatric doctor about this, I said, 'This is quite ridiculous, my wife is not going to get medication because you won't put the tablet in the end of a banana for her?' This was a cause of much concern for me and I used to get upset about it and think, 'Oh dear me, I wonder if she's been able to take her tablets.' But they don't have any nonsense at the home, they've got to do that sort of thing or nobody would take any medicine or any tablets.

In this example, why is it the case that the decision did not seem too ethically bothersome for the carer? Answering this question, we think, helps to show one way in which practice might help theory. Our suggestion is that the main thing, from the carer's perspective, was that his wife needed to get the medication; this was his ethical concern. However, he focused only on the practical issue – how to ensure that she received it – and was not concerned that there might be ethical objections to *how* she received it because his ethical concern was that she *should* receive it. Having made this ethical judgement, all that was left was a purely practical problem.

There is a similarity here, too, between the moral theories and the ethical approaches that entail the person who is engaged as an actor in the drama, and those theories and approaches that seem detached, which hold out the promise of an objective decision being made from the outside. One answer to the quandary is that ethical decisions are simply decisions that have to be made. They are decisions in the world, like any other decisions, with which we are engaged. They require that the relevant facts are known. Values and legal frameworks come into ethical dilemmas in clinical practice, as we have seen; but they are also relevant to many decisions in everyday life (for example, the decision to buy a house). Decisions are simply made in a practical (engaged) way: matters are faced, conflicts are weighed up.

So one answer to the question why do ethical decisions get made in practice in what might seem to be purely practical ways is that making decisions is a purely practical matter (when it comes to it), not a matter (usually) for theoretical debate. A decision is required, we act and the deed is done. In some cases the decision is so ethically trivial that no discussion is required. In other cases there may be debate (typically because values clash or are unclear), but this will often be decided in the end by procedural means (perhaps we need an independent advocate, or a second opinion, or a court). Ethical decisions are just a different type of practical decision.

Another reason why some ('routine') ethical dilemmas seem to cause so little trouble is that there is little time to dispute. Hence, clinicians have to fall back on their instincts. There is no time to hold an ethical case conference, a decision to act or not (in the case, say, of a man with severe dementia and a bowel obstruction) must be made quickly. All of this is not to say that sometimes an appeal to an outside body is unwarranted. Where there is time, it can be useful in a hospital to involve a clinical ethics committee, and some decisions will engender considerable debate within a team.[2] However, there are also occasions on which doctors just act with seemingly little debate, despite what is at stake from the ethical point of view. The decisions simply seem to drop from practice; that is, something about the practice itself leads to the decision. There is no need for intermediary discussion or debate. This tends, we might say, simply to be what we do under these circumstances. It does not feel like an ethical debate is necessary because, in this sort of context, we just act. But this takes us back to our earlier questions: is this just eclectic or random? Or is there some sort of guiding principle to our eclecticism? Well, we would argue, it is only as random as our patterns of practice. And one thing about patterns of practice is that they have a degree of fixity.

PATTERNS OF PRACTICE

So we make the decision to put up (or take down) the drip automatically, as it were, without ethical debate, because this is our practice. Under *these* circumstances we tend to do *this*.

Stated in this way it does not sound as if the notion of a pattern of practice has much going for it from the ethical point of view! It sounds as if we might think we can justify any practice, even bad practice, simply by making the assertion that the practice is standard. This is unsettling because we are so aware of the terrible things people have done in the past, which presumably they considered to be perfectly acceptable.

It is the same argument that is used against the notion of conscience. How can we justify our actions on the basis of conscience when it would appear that conscience can be so fickle? People seem to be able to bend their consciences. One thing to say immediately, therefore, about patterns of practice is that these patterns tend to be shared and are, therefore, less easy to bend. Hence, what we tend to do to people in the advanced stages of dementia typically involves others. If we take down a drip or start a medication, or simply wash someone, these are public acts that are normally pursued in some sort of public space with the cooperation of others. Accordingly, if this is true, it seems slightly more difficult to change a pattern of practice on a whim, especially if it is a practice of some importance.

Now, practice can go awry. There have been scandals involving individual clinicians and institutions. Such scandals have often occurred when the person or institution has become isolated. Once the scrutiny of others is brought to bear, people have to alter practice, or bad practice tends to become known. So, one important feature of patterns of practice is that they are essentially public. This helps to explain the automatic nature of some ethical decisions: they can be just part of a well-embedded pattern of practice.

To be clear, we are not arguing that the fact something is a pattern of practice makes it right! A doctor whose practice is to go about killing his elderly female patients cannot claim that this is justified because it is his practice. Nor could the manager of a home argue that tying her demented patients into their beds was morally justified on the grounds that it was the practice of the home. The doctor and the manager might appeal to patterns of practice, but the arguments against them would (in one way or another) also be appealing to broader patterns of practice against which these idiosyncratic practices would appear appropriately grim.

The question is, what makes a particular pattern of practice morally right or wrong? To answer this we need to consider what goes to make up a pattern of practice and how a particular pattern of practice might be acquired. Patterns of practice involve, potentially, a huge array of components. There will be physical practices, from handling to performing investigations. There are psychological aspects to practice, for instance to do with the carer's approach to the person. The social setting is also enormously relevant to how the pattern of practice is pursued. Then there are the moral and spiritual components to practice: the beliefs of the person involved and of the formal or informal carer. Many practices (especially non-trivial practices) are likely to have a degree of complexity.

How are complex patterns of practice acquired? Well, by training and education and by practise. We tend to do things *this* way because we have been brought up to do so. This is true whether we are talking about saying 'hello' to someone in the corridor, or whether we are talking about checking the urine when someone suddenly becomes confused. We have been 'brought up' to do both things. Such reactions or responses have become automatic (no need to deliberate too much). They have become for us akin to inner dispositions: we are naturally prone to be polite to people we pass in corridors and to check the urine in someone who might have a delirium. These are (what we might call) the virtues of practice. We should remember that the virtues themselves require education and training. But once we have them we tend to act in such and such a way: we tend to be brave once we have the virtue of bravery. So too, we are going to act in such and such a way when faced by a particular circumstance in looking after someone with dementia, because this is how we have been educated and trained to act.

We still have not answered the question of what makes a particular pattern of practice right or wrong. However, we have seen that education and training and experience are important. So then the questions should be: are our patterns of practice in keeping with our education and training? And what is morally appropriate education and training?

The first question gives us very good guidance in terms of how to judge patterns of practice. Let us presume that there is a standard way to transfer someone who is immobile from a chair into a bath. This standard pattern of practice, we can presume, will involve (among other things) considerations of safety, both with respect to the person being moved and to the movers, and considerations of dignity. It is worth noting that in itself this is an example of how an act involves both practical matters of fact (to do with the physical business of lifting) and principles relating to values (to do with respect for the person's feelings of modesty). We are presuming that the standard way of doing this is well established as a pattern of practice. Now, if a nurse starts to use a non-standard way to transfer someone, there is an immediate question. Given that the standard pattern of practice involved considering both safety and dignity, why has the nurse deviated from how he or she has been trained? It may be that the deviation is gratuitous: there is no particular reason for it except that the nurse finds it more convenient. Instantly, therefore, there is an ethical worry. Perhaps the nurse is now putting patients and staff at risk of harm and perhaps the nurse has become callous (through burnout, for example) and no longer cares about patients' dignity. The deviation from the standard pattern of practice is enough to raise alarm bells.

Equally, however, it might be that the nurse, with many years of experience, has started to see another way of performing the transfer that does the job just as well but which is even better at preserving the person's dignity, while still keeping him or her safe. That is to say, it is perfectly possible to develop a new pattern of practice requiring that people should now be educated and trained differently. Of course, having developed this new way, the nurse should follow established patterns of practice concerning such things. In other words, the nurse should discuss matters with other staff (the occupational therapist, the physiotherapist) and involve managers in the process of modifying protocols. If the new practice is really much better, it should be publicized; perhaps it will require research.

So education and training are vital to patterns of practice: where patterns of practice deviate from the norm, there must be a reason. To deviate is not necessarily to act badly; it may be to act better on the basis of experience.

Malcolm, a man whose wife had dementia, reported a difficulty he experienced with his local hospital. The practice, possibly generally good, was to ask questions directly of the patient; but in Malcolm's case this resulted in poor information being given:

> I think perhaps the most difficult thing there is that none of the hospitals appear to be geared up, geared up perhaps is overstating what I mean, but understanding of people with any form of dementia...

And certainly on several occasions when my wife was being asked questions, questions which the person asking wouldn't know whether the answers were right or wrong, I was there and, knowing it was my wife, I knew they were wrong. But I found that they were pretty reluctant to actually talk to me. And on several occasions I had to say, 'That is *not* the situation between my wife and me.'

For example, they were asking my wife if she had sex and she said, 'Yes, regularly.' I knew full well that we hadn't had any sex for a number of years. I *knew* it was the wrong answer. But the person asking the questions wouldn't know that it was a right or wrong answer.

So I think that, and indeed I did make one recommendation to one consultant that we saw that it might not be a bad idea to have a set of questions for the carer, if they're a close carer, not necessarily the same questions that they were asking the person with dementia, *but* asking if the carer had experienced any behavioural changes...

And I did suggest that it might not be a bad idea to ask the carer questions as well, I am sure that the carer can give a lot of information about the changes because they're the one that's seeing and experiencing the changes that are taking place, which could perhaps help earlier with a diagnosis.

The pattern of practice of the hospital here has very clear merits: it is important to talk and listen to the person with dementia. However, Malcolm is suggesting that the pattern of practice needs to be developed to involve listening to the family carer, which in this case would have provided more accurate information and insight into the situation.

BEING INFORMED AND OPEN TO CORRECTION

The second question we identified concerned whether we could say that the education and training that underpinned a particular pattern of practice was itself right. It could, after all, be that people are being taught to behave in ways that are morally unacceptable and we simply take the patterns of practice that result as the norm.

We recalled previously the worries about conscience being too fickle. We have argued that patterns of practice are more objective or fixed because they are (at least potentially) public. In a sense our observations about what might enable us to say that the particular education and training is moral mirrors the point in Chapter 1 about conscience. There we argued that conscience must be informed. There are two aspects to this: first, it must be genuinely informed; second, it must be open to correction. To be genuinely informed means that the person must actually have been instructed about the relevant issues. This instruction might take place in various ways (for instance by teaching, reading, or by example). The second point was that a conscience that never considered the possibility that it might be wrong would be in danger of not being properly informed. It might, indeed, be the case that the conscience was perfectly correct on whatever the point was, but a person's conscience would become better informed by considering alternatives.

Stanley was asked about whether there had been any turning points in his time caring for his wife, who had mild dementia, where he had learnt anything that had changed how he thought, felt or acted in his caring role:

> Yes, about twelve months ago I think there were two things that happened. We had a visit, at a time when my wife was going through a period of intense depression, which I could not lift her out of during last August, and we

had a wonderful friend who came to stay a few days. A lovely woman, a great, great personal friend who'd been a Samaritan, a very wise woman and it was talking to her that was one thing that made me realize that I was approaching this in the wrong way, not that she would ever dream of telling you that, but it just became clear.

Plus, I also read a book by Frena Gray-Davidson. Her approach is that the kind of clinical, medical approach to dementia is in itself inadequate and really the model must be one about interpersonal relationships and love and absolutely love without any kind of inhibitions at all and so on. That sounds rather 'waffly' I know but it did have a big effect on me and I realized that neither of us were getting any joy out of the way I was doing things. So I kind of made a solemn vow to myself that I'm never going to start blaming my wife for anything, I'm never going to get angry if I can possibly help it because any actions, anything she says or does, is not her but it's the illness.

I try to make sure that everything we do, there's some pleasure in it, some laughter and something…if it's just preparing breakfast we both try to do it in a way which kind of makes it a special occasion…it took me a year to realize that I wasn't on the right lines, it was a duty, a grim duty rather than, you know, this is my purpose for the next part of my life and it's just as worthwhile and just as interesting in a way as my past career and other things that I've done. So we are getting quite a lot of satisfaction and pleasure out of life which I hadn't ever thought would happen.

What we see here is a change of heart, which occurred because Stanley was led by the visit of his friend and by his reading to think afresh. And, of course, to be led in such a way is to be educated (because the Latin word *educare* means to lead or draw out). In our education and training, if we are to engender moral patterns of practice, we need genuine instruction and we need to be open to correction. If we are educators or trainers we cannot, therefore, simply state that we know what is best for those we educate and train without actually having received ourselves a moral education. This does not mean that we must have sat and read moral philosophy textbooks, but the learning from such textbooks must have been passed on to us somehow (perhaps only by an apprenticeship to someone who had acquired the relevant education), even if we do not recognize it as such. Furthermore, we should be open to the possibility of correction and new knowledge, which will sometimes come from theoreticians, but sometimes from practitioners.

This leads to some mundane conclusions. It means we should be in favour of things such as 'continuing professional development'. However bureaucratically tedious this might sometimes seem, by placing ourselves open to new ideas we help to ensure that our patterns of practice are up to date. Similarly, inspections and audits help to ensure that our patterns of practice are in accord with more general norms. But, of course, the inspection and audit process is itself a pattern of practice that stands in need of justification! What is important is that there needs to be coherence between patterns of practice. To lack this coherence is to be like a person whose conscience pricks: there is something not quite right if we cannot square what we do here with what we do there.

So usually the pricking of conscience alerts us to the possibility that we are doing something potentially wrong. But it is not always the case that what we are doing is actually wrong. One carer talked about his feelings of guilt when he started to take dancing lessons:

When my wife went into a home I was visiting her every day but I did have a tremendous amount of free time and I could start to think in terms of a life of my own and I started to take dancing lessons and was delighted in the process.

But I felt guilty for two reasons mainly; one is I was enjoying myself when she was suffering and, two, of course I was with other ladies, something I'd tried to avoid throughout my married life! I mean obviously you come into contact with ladies working, as I did in clerical work, but my wife was a jealous person and the idea of my associating with other women, however innocently, she would have been horrified, you know.

So, you know, I never really overcame that guilt feeling; it stayed with me all the time and even after my wife died, although I carried on dancing I felt a little bit guilty.

This is an example of a conscience pricking. It is uncomfortable, of course, to feel guilty. But how does the pattern of practice that kept this carer faithful to his wife throughout their marriage square with the pattern of practice he now pursues, which includes going to dances with other women? There is no suggestion that he was being unfaithful to his wife, and he continued to visit her and care deeply about her until she died. Indeed, his previous pattern of practice (i.e. avoiding unnecessary social contact with other women) and his present practice (i.e. attending dances) were both motivated by the desire to maintain the quality of his relationship with his wife. If the aim of attending the dances had been to establish a sexual relationship with another woman, then it would have been a practice that did not cohere with his earlier pattern of practice. However, he attended the dances in order to relieve the stress that caring placed on him, even when his wife was in a nursing home. So, on the one hand, this would be an example of how the voice of conscience can be wrong; but, on the other hand, it is an example of the way in which patterns of practice provide a more objective account of how our actions should be judged.

ECLECTIC AND OPEN PRACTICE

Patterns of practice need to be genuinely informed and open to correction. In the moral sphere what can relevantly inform or correct a pattern of practice is difficult to pin down. We have already seen that education, training and experience are vital. But there will also be moral, social, cultural, legal, political and religious or spiritual inputs to our patterns of practice (see Figure 6.1).

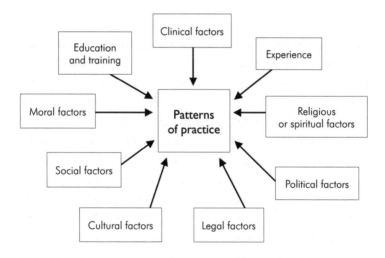

Figure 6.1 Patterns of practice

When we are making moral decisions, or decisions with a moral component, we have suggested that we often simply act in accordance with a pattern of practice. But feeding into that pattern of practice will be all sorts of influences. Our patterns of practice are ineluctably eclectic: we cannot help real-life decisions being this way, because in the real world we do need to be open to all sorts of influences. The difficulty of the decisions is often to do with being open to these various influences and the need to pick and choose between them. Sometimes we shall need to consider the consequences of an action (consequentialism), while at the same time giving weight to the importance of maintaining a relationship with the person's family (ethic of care), and it might be that taking a narrative view will help (narrative ethics), partly because it will help us to understand and decide between different perspectives (perspectivism). This is the complexity (the messiness) of the real world: there is no neat application of a moral theory here, but a need to be open and to weigh up as we pick and choose between viewpoints and approaches. All of this occurs, however, not in complete chaos with a high degree of randomness, but within patterns of practice that are essentially public, open to scrutiny and correction. Patterns of practice are also specific and concrete. They relate to particular instances, and the details and complexities are important. They must also cohere and at root must reflect our deeper instincts to become better as caring human beings. What we *are* is reflected in our patterns of practice; what we might *become* is a matter of exercising the virtues through our patterns of practice.

SUMMARY

In this chapter we have tried to answer the question about how decisions are actually made in practice. This seems like a pressing question because of the variety of approaches and theories we have previously discussed. It looked as if we

might be able to pick and choose with a worrying degree of
eclectic randomness. Rather than chaos, however, we have
found patterns of practice. We tend to act in accordance with
patterns of practice. It is within the context of a particular
pattern of practice that we are able to decide between theories
and approaches.

Patterns of practice:

- allow ethical decisions to be made as if they are
  ordinary decisions

- reflect our engagement with concrete
  circumstances

- reflect the embedding social, political, moral,
  legal, cultural and religious or spiritual culture

- have a degree of fixity because they are essentially
  public and shareable

- stem from education, training and experience

- reflect our dispositions

- need to be genuinely informed and open to
  correction or change

- require coherence.

As moral agents who engage with people with dementia and
their carers, our task is to examine our patterns of practice in
an open and informed way in order to seek coherence
between our practices and within our broader concerned way
of being in the world.

CONCLUSION

Our final reflection has been that what we become by our patterns of practice is all-important. In our dealings with people with dementia we have the potential to become more attuned to a shared humanity and the need for virtues such as patience, charity, humility, fidelity and practical wisdom. Reading (and writing) this book is also a matter of practice, reflecting an openness to ideas and reflection. But what is more important is that the period of reflection we have enjoyed and the ideas we have considered together should be put into practice in ways that benefit the lives of people with dementia and their carers.

NOTES

1. Ethical theories are dealt with in greater detail in some of the texts to which we have already referred (e.g. Gillon 1986; Beauchamp and Childress 2001; Hope *et al.* 2003). We wish to alert readers to two further examples that have been applied specifically to issues in connection with dementia: hermeneutic ethics (Widdershoven and Widdershoven-Heerding 2003; Widdershoven and Berghmans 2006) and casuistry (Louw and Hughes 2005).

2. Clinical ethics committees exist in an increasing number of hospitals or Trusts in the United Kingdom, where they serve the function of clinical ethicists in the United States. The website for the UK Clinical Ethics Network (www.ethics -network.org.uk) is an extremely useful resource.

References

Allen, F.B. and Coleman, P.G. (2006) 'Spiritual Perspectives on the Person with Dementia: Identity and Personhood.' In J.C. Hughes, S.J. Louw and S.R. Sabat (eds) *Dementia: Mind, Meaning, and the Person*, pp.205–221. Oxford: Oxford University Press.

Baldwin, C. (2005) 'Narrative, Ethics and People with Severe Mental Illness.' *Australian and New Zealand Journal of Psychiatry 39*, 1022–1029.

Baldwin, C. (2006) 'Narrative Ethics and Ethical Narratives in Dementia.' In A. Burns and B. Winblad (eds) *Severe Dementia*, 215–226. Chichester and Hoboken, NJ: Wiley.

Baldwin, C., Hope, T., Hughes, J., Jacoby, R. and Ziebland, S. (2004) 'Ethics and Dementia: The Experience of Family Carers.' *Progress in Neurology and Psychiatry 8*, 24–28.

Baldwin, C., Hope, T., Hughes, J., Jacoby, R. and Ziebland, S. (2005) *Making Difficult Decisions: The Experience of Caring for Someone with Dementia.* London: Alzheimer's Society.

Bamford, C., Lamont, S., Eccles, M., Robinson, L., May, C. and Bond, J. (2004) 'Disclosing a Diagnosis of Dementia: A Systematic Review.' *International Journal of Geriatric Psychiatry 19*, 151–169.

Beauchamp, T.L. and Childress, J.F. (2001) *Principles of Biomedical Ethics* (5th edn). Oxford: Oxford University Press.

Bond, J. and Corner, L. (2004) *Quality of Life and Older People.* Maidenhead: Open University Press.

Brooker, D. (2004) 'What is Person Centred Care?' *Reviews in Clinical Gerontology 13*, 215–222.

Cayton, H. (2006) 'From Childhood to childhood? Autonomy and Dependence through the Ages of Life.' In J.C. Hughes, S.J. Louw and S.R. Sabat (eds) *Dementia: Mind, Meaning, and the Person*, pp. 277–286. Oxford: Oxford University Press.

Council of Europe (2003) *Convention for Protection of Human Rights and Fundamental Freedoms as Amended by Protocol 11.* Strasbourg: Council of Europe.

Department of Health (2001) *Seeking Consent: Working with Older People.* London: Department of Health Publications.

Dickenson, D. and Fulford, K.W.M. (2000) *In Two Minds: A Casebook of Psychiatric Ethics.* Oxford: Oxford University Press.

Donne, J. (2000) 'Meditation XVII' in J. Carey (ed) *John Donne – The Major Works: including Songs and Sonnets and sermons.* New York: Oxford University Press. (Original work published in 1624).

Finucane, T.E., Christmas, C. and Travis, K. (1999) 'Tube Feeding in Patients with Advanced Dementia.' *Journal of the American Medical Association 282*, 1365–1370.

Fulford, K.W.M. (1991) 'The Potential of Medicine as a Resource for Philosophy.' *Theoretical Medicine 12*, 81–85.

Fulford, K.W.M. (2004) 'Facts/Values: Ten Principles of Values-based Medicine.' In J. Radden (ed) *The Philosophy of Psychiatry: A Companion*, pp.205–234. Oxford: Oxford University Press.

Gillick, M.R. (2000) 'Rethinking the Role of Tube Feeding in Patients with Advanced Dementia.' *New England Journal of Medicine 342*, 206–210.

Gilligan, C. (1982) *In a Different Voice: Psychological Theory and Women's Development.* Cambridge, MA: Harvard University Press.

Gillon, R. (1986) *Philosophical Medical Ethics.* Chichester: Wiley.

Grayling, A.C. (2001) *Wittgenstein: A Very Short Introduction.* Oxford: Oxford University Press.

Herzog, W. (Director) (1975) *The Enigma of Kaspar Hauser*. DVD. Filmverlag der Autoren, Cine International.

HMSO (1983) *Mental Health Act 1983*. London: HMSO.

Hope, T., Savulescu, J. and Hendrick, J. (2003) *Medical Ethics and Law: The Core Curriculum*. Edinburgh: Churchill Livingstone.

Hudson, W.D. (1967) *Ethical Intuitionism*. London: Macmillan.

Hughes, J.C. (2001) 'Views of the Person with Dementia.' *Journal of Medical Ethics 27*, 86–91.

Hughes, J.C. (2003) 'Quality of Life in Dementia: An Ethical and Philosophical Perspective.' *Expert Review of Pharmacoeconomics and Outcomes Research 3*, 525–534.

Hughes, J.C. (ed) (2005) *Palliative Care in Severe Dementia*. London: Quay Books.

Hughes, J.C. and Louw, S.J. (2002) 'Electronic Tagging of People with Dementia who Wander.' *British Medical Journal 325*, 847–848.

Hughes, J.C. and Louw, S.J. (2005) 'End-of-life Decisions.' In A. Burns, J. O'Brien and D. Ames (eds) *Dementia* (3rd edn), pp.239–243. London: Hodder Arnold.

Hughes, J.C., Robinson, L. and Volicer, L. (2005) 'Specialist Palliative Care in Dementia.' *British Medical Journal 330*, 57–58.

Hursthouse, R. (1999) *On Virtue Ethics*. Oxford: Oxford University Press.

Kitwood, T. (1997) *Dementia Reconsidered: The Person Comes First*. Buckingham and Philadelphia, PA: Open University Press.

Komesaroff, P.A. (1995) 'From Bioethics to Microethics: Ethical Debate and Clinical Medicine.' In P.A. Komesaroff (ed) *Troubled Bodies: Critical Perspectives on Postmodernism, Medical Ethics and the Body*, pp.62–86. Durham, NC: Duke University Press.

Lemay, E.C., Pitts, J.A. and Gordon, P. (1994) *Heidegger for Beginners*. London: Writers and Readers Publishing.

Lifton, R.J. (2000) *The Nazi Doctors: Medical Killing and the Psychology of Genocide*. New York: Basic Books.

Louw, S.J. and Hughes, J.C. (2005) 'Moral Reasoning: The Unrealized Place of Casuistry in Medical Ethics.' *International Psychogeriatrics 17*, 149–154.

McCabe, H. (2002) 'Aquinas on Good Sense.' In H. McCabe, *God Still Matters*, ed. B. Davies, pp. 152–165. London and New York: Continuum.

Moody, H.R. (1992) *Ethics in an Aging Society*. Baltimore: Johns Hopkins University Press.

Noddings, N. (1984) *Caring: A Feminine Approach to Ethics and Moral Education*. Berkeley, CA: University of California Press.

Post, S.G. (2000) *The Moral Challenge of Alzheimer Disease: Ethical Issues from Diagnosis to Dying* (2nd edn). Baltimore, MD and London: Johns Hopkins University Press.

Post, S.G. (2006) '*Respectare*: Moral Respect for the Lives of the Deeply Forgetful.' In J.C. Hughes, S.J. Louw and S.R. Sabat (eds) *Dementia: Mind, Meaning, and the Person*, pp.223–234. Oxford: Oxford University Press.

Sabat, S.R. (2001) *The Experience of Alzheimer's Disease: Life through a Tangled Veil*. Oxford and Malden, MA: Blackwell.

Sabat, S.R. (2006) 'Mind, Meaning, and Personhood in Dementia: The Effects of Positioning.' In J.C. Hughes, S.J. Louw and S.R. Sabat (eds) *Dementia: Mind, Meaning, and the Person*, pp.287–302. Oxford: Oxford University Press.

Schwartz, M.A. and Wiggins, O.P. (2004) 'Phenomenological and Hermeneutic Models: Understanding and Interpretation in Psychiatry.' In J. Radden (ed) *The Philosophy of Psychiatry: A Companion*, pp.351–363. Oxford: Oxford University Press.

Stokes, G. (2000) *Challenging Behaviour in Dementia*. Bicester: Speechmark.

Struttmann, T., Fabro, M., Romieu, G., de Roquefeuil, G., Touchon, J., Dandekar, T. and Ritchie, K. (1999) 'Quality-of-life Assessment in the Old Using the WHOQOL 100: Differences between Patients with Senile Dementia and Patients with Cancer.' *International Psychogeriatrics 11*, 273–279.

Treloar, A., Beats, B. and Philpot, M. (2000) 'A Pill in the Sandwich: Covert Medication in Food and Drink.' *Journal of the Royal Society of Medicine 93*, 408–411.

TSO (2005) *Mental Capacity Act 2005*. Norwich: The Stationery Office.

Wassermann, J. (1983) *Caspar Hauser: Enigma of a Century*. Edinburgh: Floris Books.

Widdershoven, G.A.M. and Berghmans, R.L.P. (2006) 'Meaning-making in Dementia: A Hermeneutic Perspective.' In J.C. Hughes, S.J. Louw and S.R. Sabat (eds) *Dementia: Mind, Meaning, and the Person*, pp.179–191. Oxford: Oxford University Press.

Widdershoven, G.A.M. and Widdershoven-Heerding, I. (2003) 'Understanding Dementia: A Hermeneutic Perspective.' In K.W.M. Fulford, K. Morris, J.Z. Sadler and G. Stanghellini (eds) *Nature and Narrative: An Introduction to the New Philosophy of Psychiatry*, pp.103–111. Oxford: Oxford University Press.

Subject Index

Author Index